The information and opinions expressed in this book are designed for educational purposes only. *The Longevity Source* is intended as part of an overall healthy lifestyle and for engaging in pro-active healthcare measures. It is not meant to be a substitute for medical advice, or care, when illness is encountered. Please do not use this information to diagnose or treat any health problems or illnesses without first consulting a licensed physician/Naturopath, especially if you can find an Integrative, Functional or Complimentary Alternative Medicine (CAM) Physician. Also the Optimum Health Institute, TrueNorth, Hippocrates Health Institute and Oasis of Hope are excellent choices when facing a health crisis.

Special thanks to Bruce Sherman for the cover, graphic design.
First Edition – 05/03/2015 - Hawaii

Also my utmost gratitude to all my dear friends who have contributed
their help with editing, proofreading and layout;
Lauren, Ruth, Kelly Lynn, Adam, Raven, Amber and Loraine, super Mahalo's

Likewise utmost appreciation to Nikki Spencer for the beautiful Foreword that
expresses the heart and soul of Longevity Source so well.
www.Nikki_spencer@yahoo.com

For further information and the latest updated *Resources* page please go to
www.Longevitysource.com

E-mail contact - Superfoodchef@Longevitysource.com
(Personal consultations available)

Eh Malama Pono Ekaheiau Eh

In alignment with the utmost right and highest good, may we truly care for ourselves and in so doing, be cared for and care for this Earth, and all Life, in Sacredness!

Table of Contents

1. Foreword by Nikki Spencer.....3
2. Preface.....5
3. Introduction.....10
4. Food Science and Health, 101.....20
5. Nutrigenomics, Epigenetics and Telomeres, the Core of Longevity.....20
6. Mitochondria, the Cellular Energy Powerhouse and Oxidation.....22
7. Inflamation and Chronic Illness.....23
8. A Strong Gut Microbiome, the Foundation of Health and Longevity.....24
9. Acid-Alkaline Balancing.....26
10. Enzymes and Raw Foods.....28
11. Plant Based, the Health, Environmental and Ethical Considerations.....30
12. Sustainability and a Healthy Soil Biome- the Soil-Food-Web.....36
13. GMO, Now We Know.....37
14. Mental Health, the Starving Brain and Pharmaceutical Madness.....39
15. Autism, the Gut Connection and Brain Malnourishment.....44
16. Detoxification and Common Major Toxins.....48
17. Integrative Medicine and Cleansing.....59
18. Happy, Healthy, Hormone Balance, Naturally.....62
19. Three Treasures and Tonic Herbs.....63
20. Magical Medicinal Mushrooms.....68
21. Ayurveda- The Ancient "Science of Health" from India.....70
22. Beneficial Nutrients.....74
23. Superfood Heaven Glossary.....77
24. Super Healthy Foods.....81
25. Ultra Health Adjuncts.....87
26. Skillful Lifestyle Practices.....91
27. Longevity Source Cleanse (LSC), Overview.....92
28. Cleanse Design, Objectives.....93
29. Core Cleanse Ingredients.....94
30. Longevity Source Cleanse Protocol.....101
31. Food Shopping List.....105
32. Getting Started and the 80-20 (Raw to Cooked) Diet.....106
33. Meal Planning Ideas.....107
34. Foundational Recipes.....110
35. More Recipes.....117
36. Salads and Dressings.....117
37. Dehydrated Foods.....122
38. Beverages.....124
39. Desserts.....125
40. Foundational Cooked Foods.....128
41. Resources for Sustainable and Healthy Living.....131
42. Epilogue.....140
43. Gentle World Message.....141
44. Front and Back Cover Art & Dishes- details.....143-144

Foreword
by Nikki Spencer, N.D.

Americans spend 300 billion dollars on pharmaceutical drugs a year…
This is half of what the entire world spends on pharmaceutical drugs.
SAD, SAD, SAD, SAD

Have you ever wondered "why did our government put food and drugs together into one department called the FDA (Food and Drug Administration)?" Hummm….Isn't food important enough to warrant its own office? …why does the government put food and drugs together? Because…. if you eat SAD (standard American diet), you will have SAD (standard American diseases) which will create the need for SAD (standard American drugs)… and eventually will have a SAD (standard American death). These 4 SADs create a cooperative for our diseased-based economy and this is how it works:

1. Chemical companies create pesticides and herbicides to poison the food and kill the microorganisms and bugs. This breaks down the earth's immune system and humans immune systems when they eat the food that is grown in these conditions. So the humans get sick and the earth loses its topsoil and nutrients and the microorganisms and beneficial bugs die.

2. People are told to take prescription drugs by their well-intended physicians so they can feel "better" from eating the poisoned food. We all know they never really feel better, the symptoms might be masked but a bigger problem is afoot. Big Agribusiness then adds more chemicals to the earth so more poisoned food can be grown on the increasingly depleted earth.

3. People have even more symptoms so are persuaded to take more drugs until they need to go in for surgeries or to extended care facilities. The earth continues to degrade and the corporate farmers are told they need to add more poison and chemical "nutrients" to the earth and on the cycle goes. This is how the diseased-based economy keeps moving along…

In the US $3 trillion is spent on disease management (which we ironically call health care). 75% of health care dollars are spent on diseases which are created by our lifestyles. Not much money is spent on wellness, prevention or health education. If we keep moving at this pace, by the year 2040, 100% of the federal budget will be required for Medicare and Medicaid expenses alone…Sanity?

After my own personal struggle as a child with pharmaceutical mis-treatment of severe cystic acne, I suffered a weakened immune system, candida infections, and chronic illnesses for many years until I turned to natural solutions, with excellent results.

I started studying about nutrition and lifestyle changes as well as many healing systems, and in my early 20s I obtained certificates in healing modalities such as Wise Women Herbalism, Massage, Reiki, Quantum Biofeedback and a Doctorate in Naturopathy (the study of natural medicine) by the time I was 30. I have had a healing practice and have been educating people about natural options ever since. Through the process of supplementation with vitamins, minerals, organic foods and superfoods as well as living on, with, and appreciating the land and sea, working with emotional and spiritual issues, exercise, fresh air and clean water, plus detoxification and many other things that Todd shares in *Longevity Source*, I am feeling better now in my 50s than I did in my 20s.

If we look at the words Illness and WEllness, the difference is in the I or the WE. WE need to work together with each other to get to wellness, and that is what this book is about…It is Todd's effort and the effort of many of the Functional or Integrative Medicine Doctors to get us working together in the WE. Todd has learned and now shares transformational tools that can change lives for the better. What we eat DOES matter. How we think DOES matter. We can change and age differently, gracefully, and healthfully.

I first met Vegan Chef Todd Dacey at Honaunau Bay on the Big Island of Hawaii where we would go to enjoy exquisite snorkeling and often swim with the wild dolphins. Since then Todd has advanced his repertoire and greatly expanded his education. I still go to swim in the mineral rich waters as much of possible with our ocean friends but now it is with the Raw and Superfood Vegan Chef Todd. After I purchased Todd's first book "*Vegan Inspiration*" (which is so much more than a cookbook), I was inspired and started to create many of the recipes within. I found them to be delicious and nutritious. They continue to be gratefully received at our potlucks.

Todd has been a person of great commitment and enthusiasm for creating a lifestyle that is health-driven. Not only health of the body, but of the mind and spirit. He walks his talk and is always coming up with the newest, delicious, nutrient filled creation. He is the mad scientist of superfoods…. Or I think a more accurate expression for Todd would be the BLISSFUL magician of superfoods, creating manna (life force), filled recipes wherein we can feel the life-giving essence within the dish. When you eat the food Todd prepares with Divine love and consciousness one can feel themselves reverse age. I can hardly wait to experience what he has come up with next in *The Longevity Source*!

Preface

In *The Longevity Source,* I have combined over 20 years of vegan/raw food/ superfood dietary experience and integrative healthy lifestyle exploration with the most critical, timely and helpful insights I have been blessed to receive in this last year and a half. What started last year with a one-week raw food, mind/body cleansing program at Optimum Health Institute has led to deeper research in many areas. This in-depth focus includes the exploring of an 80-20 raw to cooked diet with viewing many DVDs and online webinars by many of the leaders in health, wellness, sustainability, etc. Often, these leading pioneers revealed startling levels of widespread, serious and unnecessary health problems, as well as real solutions and fundamental ways of co-creating awareness and change.

The Longevity Source is written as a guide to share my experience, the most helpful knowledge and skills learned from these leaders, along with the time-saving and simplified superfood/raw food recipes I have been inspired to create. It is:

A. A content-rich, easily comprehensible guide to the essential knowledge needed to understand and remedy much of the current healthcare crisis.

B. A thorough insight into life-force enhancing, highly nutritious dishes that can be easily and creatively prepared, using the incredible variety, tastes and benefits of whole foods, raw foods, superfoods and tonic herbs.

C. Basic protocols for simplified detoxification and rejuvenation practices that are proven effective, yet self-pacing and comfortable.

D. Resources for the best suppliers of raw foods, superfoods, etc. plus links to the "superhero" leaders and organizations at the forefront of the health revolution, sustainability wave, and Earth transformation taking place.

~~~~

"Dean Ornish, M.D., is one of the greatest medical pioneers in the world. His research has demonstrated — for the first time — that integrative changes in diet and lifestyle can reverse heart disease, turn on health-promoting genes, slow aging, and slow or even reverse early-stage prostate cancer. Medicare and many of the largest insurance companies have made his program the first lifestyle-based approach they have ever covered. Chosen by Forbes as "one of the seven most powerful teachers in the world", Dr. Ornish's work is changing the face of medicine." -John Robbins

~~~~

I first heard the three thousand year old Taoist term "Life Cultivationist", from Ron Teeguarden of Dragon Herbs. This term is at the essence of *The Longevity Source* and states:

Life Cultivation, *"The nurturing of one's body, mind and attitude in a way that will lead to radiant health, happiness and maximized life expectancy, free from extreme degenerative diseases that afflict less diligent ones."*

~~~~

Practicing many life cultivationist choices over the last 25 years has led me to avidly exploring a wide variety of Wisdom Traditions and holistic health-wellness modalities. These explorations started with a vegan diet, and have led to a diet consisting of predominantly raw, organic, vegan, low glycemic, whole foods and superfoods. I have been an avid swimmer with wild dolphins in Hawaii since 1991, organizer of Sanskrit Kirtan chanting groups and a vegan chef caterer and author. In 2006, I published a vegan cookbook and natural health guide, *Vegan Inspiration: Whole Food Recipes for Life...*

Last summer my partner Meg and I fulfilled a long-time dream by participating in a one-week cleansing program at the Optimum Health Institute (OHI) in San Diego. OHI is a Hippocrates Institute affiliate (originally started by Ann Wigmore, the mother of wheat grass juicing) that has seen over 150,000 people go through its program in the last 30 years. Many with stage four cancer or other life threatening illnesses have come to this mind-body education center as a last resort and have turned to this wheatgrass juice plus living/raw food cleanse, education center, hoping for a miracle. Quite a few have achieved that outcome, thus creating a new life and confirming that good health is a natural state when we consume nature's pure foods.

At OHI, we experienced a live food program that eliminates meat, dairy products, and all processed and cooked foods. The cleansing and detoxification program utilizes fresh, raw, living, life-sustaining foods including sprouts, fresh vegetables, fruits, wheatgrass juice, rejuvilac, sauerkraut, seed sauces, sprouted grains, sprouted seeds, Essene crackers, vegetable juices, buckwheat and sunflower greens, gazpacho, fruit soup, raw vegetable soup, dehydrated seed and vegetable loaves, all with proper food combining.

Classes are given in exercise, relaxation, digestion and elimination, food preparation, sprouting and organic gardening. This valuable learning experience covered the proper tools to regain and maintain our natural state of wellbeing. This included nutritional, physical, mental, emotional, spiritual balance and harmony, providing the body with a healthy environment to restore itself naturally to optimum health.

We returned home to Hawaii feeling inspired and rejuvenated and started with the new 80-20 (raw to cooked) diet, which was fun and easy to transition into. I obtained a comprehensive assortment of raw food recipe books and began studying even more diligently the health benefits, philosophy, incredible variety and creativity available in the world of raw foods!

We up-leveled our long-standing raw, super-food "Magical Morning" breakfast (see "Foundational Recipes"), added a wonderful assortment of raw dishes for lunch and pretty much continued with our simple, cooked, vegan, organic, whole food dinners, interspersed with totally raw days.

My inspiration and creativity were soon blossoming, leading to the purchasing of a quality Omega food processor, high capacity blender, Green Power Juicer and Excalibur 9-drawer dehydrator. Incredible raw soups, phenomenal vegetable seed and nut pâtés, delicious, super nutritious, raw, dehydrated seed/vegetable crackers, afternoon powerful green juices, mouthwatering homemade sauerkraut and raw and regular coconut water kefirs began emerging forth from our kitchen. And yes, I was spending a little more time in the kitchen, and really enjoying the creativity and new tastes. Most importantly though, we were both finding a whole new level of energy and well-being!

I soon developed a working model for super healthy and delicious raw food preparation. This model consisted of foundational mainstay recipes I made regularly that were time efficient and could last for days. Along with some longtime favorites, I found many wonderful recipes and great health information in other books, then added my own creativity and simplified them to the core recipes and health practices I found most vital.

The new adventure continued as it became apparent there was a wealth of cutting-edge longevity, health and sustainability information widely available from an amazing variety of raw food pioneers, longevity researchers, functional medicine doctors and ecological luminaries. I became fascinated with the longevity/super nutrition and sustainability topic and began ongoing research into what the top educators were sharing.

Through online streaming webinars by a multitude of leading professionals as listed in the Resources section along with GAIAM.TV and many other books and avenues, I have found a true wealth of information. The information and wisdom from these pioneers has completely touched and opened my heart and inspired me to share this next timely level!

It soon became apparent I was receiving even more valuable information and practices than those covered in my *Vegan Inspiration* cookbook, and the inspiration to share what I was learning appeared! This was quite a surprise as I had thought that with all the great information and recipes in my previous book published in 2007, it would be the final culmination of my then, twenty years of holistic health research, professional catering experience, and cooking practice.

Yet, now I see that if *Vegan Inspiration* is like a pyramid, then *The Longevity Source* is the polished capstone on top. While *Vegan Inspiration* provides the skills to enjoy eating in a more sustainable and peaceful way, supporting good health, then *Longevity Source* provides a timely opportunity for clarifying the often complex challenges of healthy living now and the potential for a quantum leap in health and planetary evolution!

In *Longevity Source*, I have included my 80-20 recipes, many being ones I prepare most of the time and some for very special occasions! I have listed the best raw food/superfood products I know of in this book and on the *Longevitysource.com* website. The website has an ongoing, updated list of excellent resources and ways of getting significant discounts.

This book also maps out the new protocols that amazed me with their effectiveness and ones I have found supportive for years. Also included are the most transformational, ultra-effective detoxification, immune boosting and mineral plaque removing longevity protocol I know of, based on using the ultra-pure and concentrated, highest vibration superfoods and herbs from Purium superfoods. My intention is to provide a clear, simplified framework of how to get started and organized when exploring which health products, information, and dietary choices are the most cost effective and beneficial.

The Longevity Source cleanse and rejuvenation protocols thoroughly cover many of the bases needed to maintain and strengthen health. It focuses on digestion/absorption/gut health, opening detoxification pathways, dissolving mineral plaques, chelating out heavy metals, pesticide/chemical residues while supercharging the immune system to curtail virus, fungal and parasite overgrowths. It also provides bio-available and super pure, raw, superfood nutritional support. Included are supportive and delicious foundational raw recipes and cooked recipes, Ayurvedic and tonic herbal elixir drinks, medicinal mushroom and antioxidant products and super delicious, probiotic-packed, homemade coconut water Kefir and more...

The *Longevity Source* gives options for a very economical program organized to make it as easy as possible to add ingredients as experience and comfort levels develop. With the Transformational Cleanse Longevity Protocol, Twelve Pillars of Health, Skillful Lifestyle Practices, and predominant use of the Foundational

Recipes, an amazingly powerful life-enhancing program for health and wellness can be embarked upon, with truly significant, often magical results!

The research in *Longevity Source* has broadened my perspective to the incredible healing avenues available, and to the growing momentum of a beautiful worldwide network of truly caring people and organizations, cooperating together to change our society's destructive direction. Conversely, also, to the stark reality of the escalating degree of planetary crisis and unnecessary suffering of so many, especially the current younger generation.

As outlined in *Vegan Inspiration*, the massive environmental destruction and wanton animal cruelty and resulting human, mental and physical downhill health trends were epic enough. Now to embrace the sobering reality of us facing multiple, monumental planetary wide environmental/ecological crisis's along with so many in the younger generations being afflicted with escalating rates of unnecessary, runaway levels of cancer, autism, diabetes and all manner of digestive issues and food allergies. This evokes incredible sadness, a yearning for change and has been of major impetus in the writing of this book.

~~~~

"The prospect of uncovering our innermost feelings about what is happening to our world is daunting. How to confront what we scarcely dare to think? How to face such grief and fear and rage without going to pieces?"
-Joanna Macey, Positive Disintegration- Shambala Sun, Jan. 2015

~~~~

I have included much of this information, not to elicit any resentment or focus on the negative, but to graphically show how important it is to be super mindful about what affects our earth, us, our family's and loved ones' health. Also to understand and motivate choosing the avenues of sustainable living, inspired activism, diet, detoxification and rejuvenation protocols so important to our continued and improved well-being.

~~~~

"We're doing something that's utterly out of phase with our own greatness, our own beauty, and our own love. We are literally destroying the earth on which we depend for our food, for our economy, and for our lives. The effort to bring our food systems, our personal choices, our ways of life, and our definition of success back into alignment with the well-being of the whole is a tremendous challenge." -Ocean Robbins

~~~~

My deepest hope and prayer is that you and those you touch find super health and aliveness and that *The Longevity Source* is of true value to you on your path to wellbeing, health and longevity! May we all experience reaching our highest potential as we receive a fully functioning immune system, blossoming probiotic population, crystal clear intellect, and wide open heart to help fulfill our part to play in creating the world we know is possible.

May you add years to your life filled with enlightened energy, highest purpose and loving kindness for yourself, loved ones and the world around you. May this book be of value on the journey into wellness.

Many Blessings and much gratitude to Divine Source, my forever supportive partner Meg, and all the loved ones who have helped in the bringing forth of this book. Also, most gratefully to all the super hero pioneers of longevity, health and truth leading the way to a sustainable world manifesting!
Mahalo Nui Loa, Blessed Be
Superfood Vegan Chef Todd Dacey

Introduction

My prayer and intention in writing *The Longevity Source* is to provide practical protocols, beneficial insights, and the best resources to support thriving in today's world, to help make tomorrow's even better! At this time, human civilization is unsustainable and without an ecological U-turn, in a sure-fire terminal situation.

~~~~

"This created a "food bubble," a temporary and artificial expansion of the food supply the world briefly experienced in the last half of the twentieth century. What seems like man keeping up with the needs of a growing population destroys our children's means of food production. Every element of this process is unsustainable. Farmland is stripped of nutrients. Chemicals destroy the organisms needed to convert matter to topsoil. Rainforests turn into deserts, the atmosphere becomes more polluted, and aquifers are drained. Genetically modified seeds contaminate natural varieties, so native crops require excessive irrigation and chemicals to produce harvests. Food bubbles are ready to burst in many places simultaneously." -Food Democracy Now

~~~~

Due in large part to corporate greed, government corruption, and blatant shortsightedness, we have allowed a healthcare and food production system that is flagrantly inadequate. Bottom line predatory capitalism economics based on maximum corporate profit, rather than including human, environmental and animal welfare policies, are quickly leading us towards self-destruction.

"Our conversion from local, fully integrated food systems, to industrial monocultured agricultural production has brought a staggering number of side effects, many of them unanticipated. Throughout the entire food system we can trace the crisis as it manifests itself in soil erosion, poisoned ground waters, food borne illness, loss of biodiversity, inequitable social consequences, toxic chemicals in food and fiber, loss of beauty, loss of species and wildlife habitat, and myriad other environmental and social problems. To make the crisis even worse we continue to export this destructive industrial system of food production around the Earth." -Douglas Tompkins, Fatal Harvest

~~~~

The staggering increases in disease rates, especially with our children, the often harmful mistreatment/suppression of illness symptoms with pharmaceuticals, along with the world wide spread of environmental toxicities has to change for us to have a sustainable future.

~~~~

"The number 350 means climate safety. To preserve a livable planet, scientists tell us we must reduce the amount of CO2 in the atmosphere from its current level of 400 parts per million to below 350 ppm.

We believe a global grassroots movement can hold our leaders accountable to the realities of science and the principles of justice. That movement is rising from the bottom up, all over the world, and is uniting to create the solutions that will ensure a better future for us all." www.350.com

~~~~

The number of us that have been affected by the epidemic of degenerative diseases sweeping the nation is alarming. The compromised state of the food supply can be aptly termed "post-apocalyptic" by anyone with an accurate overview of what's happening. A severe nutrient deficiency has taken place with the consumption of now nutrient-deficient monocultured foods, processed food dependence, unconscious intake of refined sugar and high fructose corn syrup, GMO-related allergies, and intestinally related nutrient absorption with lack of availability issues. Consumption of these pseudo-food "anti-nutrients" drains the body's nutritional reserves, with all of the above adding to our skyrocketing healthcare crisis.

~~~~

"We eat our daily bread without being conscious of the massive loss of topsoil, diversity and farm communities involved in its production. We happily munch on hamburgers without a thought to the forests and prairie being destroyed for cattle grazing or the immense cruelty in the raising and slaughtering of the animals. Mothers continue to prod their youngsters to eat their vegetables, unaware of the

11

pesticide poisoning of our water, farm workers and wildlife that is involved in their production, not to mention the new human health and ecological risks of genetic engineering. This distancing and ignorance make us all unintentionally complicit in the eco-crimes and social devastation caused by current agriculture. In this way industrial food creates a moral as well as an environmental crisis."
-Alice Waters, Fatal Harvest

~~~~

So-called psychological illness is skyrocketing, in large part because of lifestyle factors, nutritionally starved brains, and widespread intestinal dysregularities. The Vegas nerve directly connects the gut and brain, thus intestinal health and mental health are greatly correlated. An area of real concern is the routine prescribing of psychotropic, or antidepressant drugs, using sketchy diagnostic tools. This is usually done without a second thought given to resulting dangerous side effects and the huge rate of success with detoxification and improving nutrition, gut health, diet and lifestyle factors. We now have over seventy million Americans, including over seven million youths taking these often harmful prescription drugs.

~~~~

"The interconnectedness of your gut, brain, immune, and hormonal systems is impossible to unwind. Until we begin to appreciate this complex relationship, we will not be able to prevent or intervene effectively in depression, slated to become the second-leading cause of disability in this country, within the decade."
–Kelly Brogan M.D.

~~~~

While much of the ocean life is toxically polluted or decimated, CAFOs or concentrated animal factory operations are creating health, environmental, and moral decline. While the increasing pollution from animal farms, which are producing many times more excrement than humans worsens, the effect on our nation's health of the daily eating of 24 million (over 99% of all meat sold in the US is from CAFOs) GMO fed, pharmaceutical and chemically loaded, cooked in toxic oils, unhealthy and mistreated animals and their eggs and milk adds greatly to the major healthcare, environmental and moral crisis unfolding.

~~~~

"The whole industrial model of meat production is only cheap because it externalizes the costs onto society. If factory farms and feedlots had to pay full market value for the feed crops and water they use, the price of the products would be so high that Americans would have to treat them less like a staple and more like a garnish. If factory farms had to pay their own pollution costs instead of getting taxpayers to both pick up the tab and also suffer the consequences of

the pollution, the whole model would no longer be economically viable. We need to stop subsidizing this tragic way of producing our food. And we need to stop the routine use of antibiotics in factory farms (due to such unhealthy crowded conditions) that is fueling the increasing development of superbugs resistant to our best medicines." -Jonathan Foer, EatingAnimals.com

~~~~

While gigantic multinational processed food and agricultural chemical companies prosper, (Monsanto's reported quarterly profit is 5 billion dollars) Americans are consuming one of the worst diets imaginable, leading us to becoming # 34 down on the list of healthy populations. The predatory style of processed food companies developing and marketing super addictive "hyper palatable" pseudo foods is wreaking havoc with our health.

With high levels of sugar, salt, fat and chemicals added, they are intentionally designed to be addictive. Processed food companies hire "craveability" experts to increase "heavy users"and "stomach share." As kids are preyed upon with TV ads and junk food in schools, the government subsidizes the very ingredients in these products that are leading to major healthcare issues, including skyrocketing diabetes and obesity rates.

~~~~

"Scientists have discovered that sugar is more addictive and more toxic than most of us ever imagined. And it's being added to more than three-quarters of the foods sold in the United States. A farmer can spray chemicals to kill bugs, then spray more chemicals to kill weeds, and then add chemicals to the soil… and we don't require any labels. But if a farmer wants to use an organic sticker, they have to pay a bunch of money, and fill out loads of paperwork, to prove they didn't use chemicals. All of life is on the line. Our planet's climate is in serious trouble, and industrialized agriculture is a driving force." -Food Democracy Now!

~~~~

As more and more kids suffer, the impact on the future becomes alarming. With most of the food supply being compromised with toxins and processed or genetically altered substances beyond the body's recognition, these harmful junk foods are causing skyrocketing allergic reactions, impaired gut health/leaky gut, immune disorders and a worsening spectrum of chronic illness epidemics at runaway rates. Toxin riddled clothing, beds, household cleaners, body care/beauty products, yard care and over the counter drugs are commonly used be my most Americans, adding even more challenges to overburdened systems.

~~~~

"Two out of three people contracting type 2 adult onset diabetes now are children below 16. Pediatric cancer as leading cause of death in those under 15 years of age with an escalating rate of pediatric hospitals being built. Our kids are sicker than ever and while being 30 % of the population now, they are 100% of the future. If we can't come to a consensus to protect the youngest among us, I don't know what kind of humans we think we are.

What is the hardest thing you have to deal with? "The hardest thing I have to deal with is [that] the sickest people I deal with today are youngsters. It used to be a lot easier when I began my work, because people my age and older were sick. Now it's common for me to work with teenagers and younger – or 20-year-olds and 30-year-olds – with major, major, major disease. And we're getting calls on a daily basis from the youth and their parents talking about catastrophic concerns these people have. We are out of control, totally out of control."
Dr. Brian Clement

~~~~

Most doctors have genuinely good intentions and often offer excellent lifesaving skills with acute care and some health situations. Conversely, a vast majority are deficient in the fundamental health principles necessary to actually positively help the majority of their chronically ill patients. By not being educated to, or ignoring functional medicine, needed nutritional, dietary and lifestyle improvement protocols, many patients are entangled in a complex web of pharmaceutical medicines, misinformation, and invasive, unhelpful procedures. I would estimate up to 90% of chronic illness that's responded to by the medical profession with the standard model of pharmaceuticals and various surgeries would have a quantumly improved outcome following basic diet and lifestyle remediation's.

This convoluted situation seems to evade resolution partly because of the amazingly helpful lifesaving abilities and technology that are also a part of modern medicine. The tremendous good of many skillful and caring professionals so many have received benefit from, including me, cannot be negated, while the shortcomings are acknowledged and resolved!

~~~~

"Nevertheless, CAD (Coronary Artery Disease) remains the number one killer of women and men in this country. Thousands of stable patients having stents experience no reduction in major cardiac events. While drugs have some effects on disease initiation and progression, these interventions do not address disease causation. Not surprisingly, most patients experience disease progression, more drugs, more imaging, repeat interventions, progressive disability, and, too often, death from a disease of western malnutrition, the cause of which has been largely left untreated." -Caldwell Esselyn MD

I recently heard Mark Hyman relating an account of a young man who had been in and out of hospitals for years with debilitating, serious skin conditions, rashes etc. Hospital and Dr. costs had totaled almost half a million dollars. As Mark used a protocol, based on integrative and functional medicine, this fortunate young man was well on his way to complete recovery in 3 weeks for a fraction of the cost and side effects of usual medical treatment. How many more of our population/youth are caught up in these defective treatment practices?

~~~~

"The practice of medicine as we know it is not actually designed to support the health of people. It's really designed to diagnose and treat disease, primarily with drugs and surgery. We might think that a doctor would be someone who would know about preventing disease and promoting health. But in fact, compared to others, our medical doctors live shorter lives. They have a higher rate of drug addiction, and they have more heart disease. They aren't examples of health, because they haven't learned the principles of healthy living.

Their education has taught them a great deal about drugs, surgery, treatments, and procedures. But they've been taught little to nothing about the practices and principles that actually prevent disease in the first place. Doctors are working in a system that pushes them really hard, and they are usually so overworked that they don't have time to investigate on their own. They haven't been taught, and generally don't learn, much if anything about prevention." -Dean Ornish MD

~~~~

Stressful lifestyles fueled by caffeine, chemicalized, sugared, processed and fast foods and an onslaught of EMF generating media devices, combined with nonstop negative media programming have further added to health issues, psychological disturbances and a spiritual disconnection from ourselves.

~~~~

"If you think it's bad and frightening at this stage, at the beginning of the 21st century, you wait as we march forward with no control over corporate greed because the disease rate is so skyrocketing at this point it's frightening, where diabetes is so rampant, autism is so rampant, cancer is the second killer of children. Children are having heart attacks in their teens at this point. The people who are supposed to be protecting the citizens of a country, and this is all countries around the world, turn their blind eye to this. What kind of people are we and how can they sleep at night? But let me tell you, it's going to come back because the cost to the governments is going to be so overwhelming. It's going to be a tsunami, a tidal wave of impossibility to run any nation in the world with that many millions and millions of sick citizens." -Brian Clement

With every crisis, however, there is great opportunity, a great awakening is taking place and a beautiful future is possible – perhaps one that is even more amazing than we can imagine. A shift in consciousness from separateness to connection, from competition to cooperation is what's needed most to move toward manifesting our full potential. The future of our species and our planet is calling for us to have a fundamental transformation into a "life economy."

This "Triple Bottom Line" life economy policy takes into account ecological, social, and economic impacts, enhancing quality of life for the entire planet. By having economy and technology become a subsidiary of ecology, whole new systems, structures and consciousness can develop. By accounting for ecological/health impact, cleanest becomes cheapest. In conscious capitalism, when there is accountability and responsibility for ecological impact, then a fundamental and beautiful healing relationship with the Earth unfolds!

~~~~

"Given the need to simultaneously stabilize climate, stabilize population, eradicate poverty, and restore the earth's natural systems, our early twenty-first-century civilization is facing challenges that have no precedent. Rising to any one of these challenges would be taxing, but we have gotten ourselves into a situation where we have to effectively respond to each of them at the same time, given their mutual interdependence. And food security depends on reaching all four goals. There is no middle ground with Plan B."
-World Business Academy (Download of Plan B available! (www.worldbusiness.org)

~~~~

By being involved in and supporting triple bottom line business (people, planet, profit) we are supporting the companies whose purpose, mission, and driving force is not just about making money, it's first about serving the greater good. By being an unstoppable force for good, we experience being in the highest integrity with who we really are!

~~~~

"At Center for Food Safety, our mission is to protect the public health and environment from the harmful impacts of the current industrial food system, and instead nurture a sustainable food future. Thus we define "food safety" broadly and holistically, meaning food that is not just safe to eat, but also, among other things, environmentally sustainable, biologically diverse, family-scale, local, climate friendly, socially just, humane, nutritious, transparent, and properly labeled. For us, the vital U.S. Department of Agriculture (USDA) organic standard should be the floor, not the ceiling." -Center for Food Safety (CFS)

It's high time for this heroic and important shift to a life-affirming economy based on full disclosure of true ecological impact costs. To shift from this industrial, toxic food culture model to a "true-cost economy", toxicity and pollution externalities are internalized making it unprofitable to harm the planet or people.

~~~~

"Switching to a plant-based diet, we could reduce petroleum usage and imports enormously, and slash the amount of hydrocarbons and carbon dioxide that contribute to air pollution and the largest cause of global warming. We could save hundreds of billions of dollars per year in medical, drug, and insurance expenses, which could boost personal savings and thus reinvigorate the economy, providing fresh funds for creative projects and environmental restoration. Desolate mono-cropped fields devoted to livestock feed could be planted with trees, bringing back forests, streams and wildlife. Marine ecosystems could rebuild, rain forests could begin healing, and with our demand for resources of all kinds dramatically reduced, environmental and military tension could ease." -Will Tuttle

~~~~

A beautiful wave of change is gaining momentum in the midst of our looming global crisis. I am so grateful for the uplifting world of so many great spiritual, environmental and natural health leaders that have emerged, synergistically cooperating to help in the quantum shift and to spread the message of real change. A wonderful selection of resources, organizations and people are quoted throughout this book and listed in the resource section for further exploration!

The beguiling pictures of our own decline make it so important for those who have awareness to help transform this. With knives and forks we can dig ourselves out of a grave into a thriving future. Our choice at meal time is a fundamental and paramount part of how we change the world. What we eat is intimate, political, and cultural.

~~~~

"Large-scale industrialized food production is wreaking havoc on our forests, topsoil, air, water, and climate. Farm animals are being treated with tremendous cruelty, and farm workers are often exploited. Genetically engineered "frankenfoods" are being released, without adequate testing, into the food supply on a vast scale. Meanwhile, people are eating more and more artificial food—and getting fatter and sicker. In fact, more people are chronically ill today than at any time in the history of the world." –Center for Food Safety

~~~~

When we understand the multi-dimensional consequences of our food and lifestyle choices, we can see how our choices directly affect our own health, the environment, world hunger, our relationships, consciousness, genetics, direction of society and world more than almost anything else!

~~~~

"As many of us as possible need to undergo a massive transformation of consciousness and to find the sacred passion to act from this consciousness in every arena and on every level of reality. It is my deepest belief that only Sacred Activism – the fusion of the deepest mystical knowledge, peace, strength, and stamina with calm focused and radical action – can possibly be of use now."
-Andrew Harvey, Sacred Activism

~~~~

To help ourselves, our children and fellow beings, its paramount to add our brilliance to the expanding wave of health pioneers, eco activists and wellness leaders actually changing the direction we are going! We are in this together and only together can we create the grace and miracles to evolve and thrive as one community! At this time it's profoundly significant to be a responsible and caring member of the extended community to which we belong, the global human family, and the exquisite ecosystem we call Earth.

~~~~

"Thousands of young Americans have dedicated themselves to reforming the food chain, from field to table, and of all the programs that have emerged to channel that energy and idealism, FoodCorps is the most inspiring."-M. Pollan
***Our Mission**, together with communities, FoodCorps serves to connect kids to healthy food in school.*
***Our Vision**, we are creating a future in which all our nation's children— regardless of class, race, or geography—know what healthy food is, care where it comes from, and eat it every day. Through our work, future generations will grow up to lead healthier and more productive lives.*
***Our Values**, we believe big things are possible. We are committed to building a solution that matches the vast scale of the problem, and to approaching and evaluating our work with a rigor that makes our ambitious vision a reality.*
***We believe** healthy food has healthy roots. So the food we serve is truly nourishing, we strive for it to be good for the people who grow, harvest, prepare and eat it and for the lands and waters where it is produced."* www.foodcorps.org

~~~~

"Also remember that although things seem overwhelming and like lost and hopeless at this point it's not, because what I've seen in my lifetime is when people are up against the wall and everything seems like it's coming to an end that humanity will rebound. We will take back our life, take back our health and we will start to direct our destiny rather than have it directed for us."-B. Clement

How may we create a viable future for ourselves, our families, communities and Humanity as a whole? All each and every one of us can do is to keep up-leveling ourselves in every way possible, tuning into the Divine guidance within and connecting with our fellow Beloved beings committed to making a difference.

~~~~

"More economic theories and external controls will not solve this deepening crisis. Only when our hearts experience the Divine reality that there is only one Human Family, one Human Race, and that all Mother Earth is the common spiritual heritage of all beings, will we be able to develop a global economic system that is life preserving and life sustaining." -Dan Lane

~~~~

I feel certain there is a miracle possible, an outcome of Amazing Grace that spontaneously arises from the coherent, resonant, love and passion of our ever increasing wave of change, generating a unified field that creates the space for a New Earth. May we all find the ways to embody that resonant field of dreams to live in our Heaven on Earth. Mahalo and Blessings, Superfood Chef Todd

~~~~

"As a wise Elder once told me, whenever we make economic gain on the weakness of others or unfairly exploit others for our own selfish purposes, we will pay a very high price. In essence, the hurt of one is the hurt of all, and the honor of one is the honor of all." It's only a matter of time when global economic convulsions will impact every nation on Mother Earth. The spiritual reality that must be realized is that the Old World Order based in greed, materialism and economic elitism is no longer able to meet the needs of the growing Spiritual Consciousness of the Peoples of Mother Earth. Only by providing positive alternatives to the destructive and inharmonious patterns of living will we rebuild our Families, Communities and Nations." -Native American Elder, Dan Lane

~~~~

"We are called on only to be politically active and to make lifestyle changes The choice is ours—yours and mine. We can stay with business as usual (Plan A) and preside over an economy that continues to destroy its natural support systems until it destroys itself, or we can adopt Plan B (ASAP) and be the generation that changes direction, moving the world onto a path of sustained progress. The choice will be made by our generation, but it will affect life on earth for all generations to come." -Lester Brown, World Business Academy

~~~~

Food Science and Health 101

The multi-dimensional repurcussions, both personally and planetarily, of our dietary choices form the most relevant criteria for discerning healthy foods. If we want to have any chance, whatsoever, in having a viable future and a healthier population it is of the utmost importance, especially for our youth, to be educated about and understand sustainability, the soil-food-web and the foundational, most important "physiological and sociological consequences" of our food choices.

The first consideration is based on clearly understanding the realities of functional medicine, how our bodies have varying responses to the different ingredients in dietary choices - the effects on our physiological and neurological well-being. Environmental and plant health, due to soil and growing conditions, (the soil-food-web) is likewise of utmost importance along with taking into account production ethics, based on a "true cost" economy and the "triple bottom line" priorities of responsible businesses; people, planet, then profit.

What we put at the end of our fork is more powerful medicine, in most cases, than anything in a pill bottle. Food is the most powerful medicine available to heal chronic disease, which will account for over 50 million deaths and cost the global economy $47 trillion by 2030. The most powerful tool we have to change our brain and our health is our fork. Food is not just calories or energy. Food contains information that talks to our genes, turning them on or off and affecting their function moment to moment. By consuming a balanced, unprocessed diet that's full of life force- raw, sustainably-organically grown foods, especially fruits and vegetables, our body's will acquire the essential nutrients and antioxidants required to achieve or maintain optimal health.

Nutrigenomics, Epigenetics and Telomeres, the Core of Longevity

Food is the fastest acting and most powerful medicine we can take to change our life. This is called nutrigenomics and is research focusing on identifying and understanding molecular-level interaction between nutrients and other dietary bioactives with the genome. Think of our genes as the software that runs everything in our body. Just like our computer software, our genes only do what we instruct them to do with the stroke of our keyboard. The foods we eat are the keystrokes that send messages to our genes telling our DNA what to do— switching on or off genes that lead to health or disease. What we eat programs our body with messages of health or illness.

Beyond simply being a mechanism for conveying calories, food is a source of special ingredients than can prevent and treat disease and transform our health. These are called phytonutrients – special plant chemicals that are not calories, protein, fat, carbohydrates, vitamins and minerals, but special molecules that interact with our biology, special molecules that act like switches on our DNA to heal our body. This entirely new branch of biological science is called epigenetics and is the science of how our DNA changes continuously based on our diet-lifestyle, emotions, and environment. We have much more control over your body, mind, and brain than we might think.

~~~~

"The more you change your diet and lifestyle, the more you improve in virtually every way we can measure, whether it is your heart disease improving, your PSA coming down,(A test for a prostrate produced enzyme that at elevated levels shows increased cancer risk) or your gene expression changing. We found that over 500 genes were changed in just three months, with the up-regulating or turning on of genes that prevent disease, and down regulating or turning off of genes that help promote disease. Particularly what are called the RAS oncogenes that promote cancers of the prostate, breast, and colon were down regulated. These processes are much more dynamic than anyone had realized. The more we look, the more we find." -Dean Ornish

~~~~

Phytonutrients, also referred to as phytochemicals ("phyto" meaning "plant"), are the chemical compounds that give fruits, vegetables, grains, nuts, teas, legumes and spices their color. The mechanisms of action for many of these plant chemicals include powerful antioxidant, anti-inflammatory, anti-viral and anti-bacterial modulations. Consuming these plant compounds can have extraordinarily positive effects on different areas of the body. Major group classifications include;

Carotenoids like beta-carotene, lutein, zeaxanthin and lycopene found in carrots, spinach, tomato etc.), Phenolics and Flavenoids like ellagic acid, quercetin, luteolin, hesperitin and genisten are found in apples, berries, citrus, green tea, olives, grapes, etc). Glucosinolates found in cabbage, broccoli, cauliflower, radish etc.) Resveratrol found in red & purple grapes, red wine, blueberries and cranberries. Tanins found in pomegranate, persimmon, nuts, lentils and green tea. When we consume these plant compounds, many health benefits are conferred to us.

"Everytime you eat or drink you are either feeding disease or fighting it".
Food Revolution Network

A newly emerging science is the study of neuroplasticity, or brain plasticity—which means, we are literally reforming our brain with each passing day. Our brain possesses the remarkable ability to reorganize pathways, create new connections and, in some cases, even create new neurons throughout our entire lifetime. Our brain is not "programmed" to shrink and fail as we age. Our brain's plasticity is controlled by our diet and lifestyle choices. The foods we eat (especially anti-inflamatory and antioxidant rich foods that counter oxidative rust as in Alzheimers), exercise, emotional states, sleep patterns, and our level of stress—all of these factors influence our brain from one moment to the next.

Another major longevity factor scientists have found is the ticking biological "clock" that offers clues on aging and longevity: telomeres. At both ends of every DNA strand in a human cell is a telomere. Telomeres prevent chromosomes from becoming frayed, fusing into rings, or binding with other DNA. It can be thought of as the protective cap that protects shoelaces from unraveling. Based on numerous human studies showing the association of shortened telomeres with premature aging, the health of the DNA's telomeres may mean living life to its fullest with a feeling of youthful health and vibrancy or not.

As part of our body's normal aging process, each time a cell divides the telomere ends in DNA get shorter. Add oxidative stress to the mix and telomeres shorten even more rapidly. Oxidative stress is the effect of destructive reactions in the body's cells caused by too many free radicals or atoms/molecules that have unpaired electrons. Free radicals come from environmental toxins, such as pollution, chemicals, drugs and radiation, and naturally occur in our own body, with exercise.

When telomeres get short, cells are unable to divide (or reproduce) and simply die. Eventually, this instability leads to tissue breakdown, cell replication abnormalities and premature aging. Antioxidants fight free radicals and stem the causes of oxidative stress, and many lifestyle factors also help to reduce oxidative stress and its effects on our telomeres.

Mitochondria, the cellular energy powerhouse and oxidation

We have over 100,000 trillion Mitochondria, the energy powerhouse of the cell, in the body. These powerhouses each contain 17,000 little assembly lines for making ATP, our major fuel. They use over ninety percent of the oxygen we breathe. They take up forty percent of the space inside the heart cells.

These little energy factories are sensitive to "insults." They are not well protected and easily damaged by toxins, infections, allergens, and stress. But the biggest insult over time is eating too much food, too many "empty calories." When the

22

food is burned or metabolized with oxygen in the mitochondria, waste is produced in the form of free radicals that create a chain reaction of rusting or oxidation.

Unless we have enough antioxidants in our diet, or we make enough in our body, we can't protect ourselves from the damage to our mitochondria. Free radicals are linked to over 60 different diseases. If our body does not get adequate protection, free radicals can become rampant, causing cells to perform poorly. This can lead to tissue degradation and the risk of diseases. Free radicals can severely affect our DNA by disrupting the duplication of DNA, interfering with DNA maintenance and altering its structure by reacting with the DNA bases.

So when we eat empty calories, meaning sugar, flour, and processed foods that don't have the antioxidant levels of colorful plant foods like fruits and vegetables, we produce too many free radicals that destroy our mitochondria and produce fatigue, metabolic burnout, and all the diseases of aging.

Inflammation and Chronic Illness

Our immune system attacks anything in our body that it recognizes as foreign— such as an invading microbe, plant pollen, or chemical. The process is called inflammation. Intermittent bouts of inflammation directed at truly threatening invaders protect our health. However, sometimes inflammation persists, day in and day out, even when we are not threatened by a foreign invader. That's when inflammation can become an enemy.

Hidden inflammation, run amok, is at the root of all chronic illness we experience — conditions like heart disease, obesity, diabetes, dementia, depression, cancer, and even autism. We may feel healthy, but if this inflammation is raging inside of us, then we are in trouble. The real concern is the chronic inflammation that slowly destroys organs and the ability to function optimally leading to rapid aging.

It's important to realize that dietary components can either prevent or trigger inflammation from taking root in our body, and processed foods do the latter, with pro-inflammatory ingredients like high fructose corn syrup, GMO soy, processed vegetable oils (trans fats), and other chemical additives. A diet high in processed and cooked foods, particularly those made from white flour, sugar, factory farm dairy and meats, will push the body towards an inflammatory state.

~~~~

"Any given gene is not in a static "on" or "off" position. You may be a carrier of a gene that never gets expressed, simply because you never supply the required environment to turn it on. As neurologist David Perlmutter explains:

"We interact with our genome every moment of our lives, and we can do so very, very positively. Keeping your blood sugar low is very positive in terms of allowing the genes to express reduced inflammation, which increase the production of life-giving antioxidants. So that's rule number one: You can change your genetic destiny." -Dr. Mercola

A Strong Gut Microbiome- the Foundation of Health and Longevity

A healthy intestinal probiotic (microbiota) population is critical for wellness and living on this planet. A compromised internal digestive terrain of the body- the "gut biome" is a serious condition that must be overcome. To live longer and stronger we have to do our best to have a strong and healthy immune system through a hardy inner eco-system.

~~~~

"In our modern day American food culture, however, we're looking down an increasingly long road of less-than-optimal food resources. Highly processed and highly palatable "high-convenience" foods may make the day go a little easier at dinner time, but it certainly isn't doing our gut any favors. Stripped of nutrients, enzymes, and minerals, only to be replaced with non-organic compounds (to extend shelf life, etc.) we see more and more food allergies and sensitivities popping up than there ever were in our parents or grandparents generation.

Couple that with the over-zealous use of antibiotics and over-the-counter medicines, not to mention the amount of antibiotics used in conventional meat and dairy production, and we're looking at a perfect storm when it comes to a less-than optimal environment inside our human microbiome."
-Marc David, Psychologyofeating.com

~~~~

The digestive track absorbs and breaks down food for energy and makes important substances that protect against pathogens. Healthy intestinal bacteria weigh 3-4 lbs. (often called the undiscovered organ) and are defined as: "Probiotic-for life, a microbe that protects and benefits its host and prevents disease." It is the ultimate enzyme, best antioxidant, powerful detoxifier, energy producer and manager. Seventy percent of the immune system is in the gut!

~~~~

"When you eat or drink foods that have been fermented, the beneficial microflora multiplies the nutrients in those fermented foods by hundreds of times. They also improve your ability to absorb nutrients by acting like digestive enzymes. This is important because as we age our body produces less digestive enzymes and our ability to digest nutrients - including those nutrients important for brain health -

becomes quite poor. Since microflora also help nurture and protect the gut wall barrier they create a healthy intestinal lining - also essential to ensure proper absorption of nutrients." -Donna Gates, The Body ecology Diet

~~~~

Our intestinal organisms, or microbiome, participate in a wide variety of bodily systems, including immunity, detoxification, inflammation, neurotransmitter and vitamin production, nutrient absorption, whether we feel hungry or full, and how we utilize carbohydrates and fat. All of these processes factor into whether we experience chronic health problems like allergies, asthma, ADHD, cancer, type 2Diabetes or dementia.

In the latest research we now know that our microbiome also affects mood, libido, and even our perceptions of the world and the clarity of our thoughts. A dysfunctional microbiome could be at the root of headaches, anxiety, inability to concentrate, or negative outlook on life.

~~~~

To restore gut health and balance, from a "disbiotic" environment, it's important to eliminate bad yeast and other opportunistic, parasitic organisms, and then restore friendly bacteria and digestion. Friendly bacteria and beneficial yeast and Kefir cultures are essential to a wide range of bodily functions. They help white blood cells fight disease, control putrefactive bacteria in the intestines, provide important nutrients for building blood, assist digestion, protect intestinal mucosa, prevent diarrhea and constipation, and manufacture B vitamins, especially B12.

When samples of high-quality, fermented organic vegetables made with starter cultures is tested, a typical serving (about two to three ounces) can contain not only 10 trillion beneficial bacteria, it also can have 500 mcg of vitamin K2, which we now know is a vital co-nutrient to both vitamin D and calcium. Most high-quality probiotic supplements supply only a fraction of the beneficial bacteria found in homemade, fermented organic veggies, so it's the most economical route to optimal gut health as well.

~~~~

"Lactobacillus kefir alone was found to fight the toxins produced by Clostridium difficile, a bacterium that contributes to chronic and sometimes deadly diarrhea. Because C. difficile is increasingly resistant to antibiotics, C. difficile infection is life threatening." -Donna Gates, The Body Ecology Diet

Healthy bacteria in our gut reduces inflammation. The entire immune system (and our body) is protected from the toxic environment in the gut by a layer only one cell thick. This thin layer covers a surface area the size of a tennis court—yet it's basically containing a sewer. If that barrier is damaged, sickness and creating an overactive immune system result (Auto-immune), producing inflammation throughout the body.

This important microbial balance can be wiped out by stress, sugar, gluten foods, antibiotics, etc. This results in a host of problems including colon cancer, malnutrition, constipation, obesity (probiotics regulate appetite), infections, sugar cravings and even negatively effecting behavior and brain function. As above so below, as the gut sends chemical messengers to the brain, via the Vegas nerve, directly affecting mood and cognition. Often this functional issue is mislabeled as depression and erroneously treated with pharmaceutical drugs.

Yeast infections are dangerous! They produce toxins that challenge the immune system, poison our bloodstream, affecting energy and mood. Yeast damages the pancreas and adheres to the digestive track. It soon begins to break through and causes leaky gut, spreading throughout the body. It can form bio-films where other unwelcome guests proliferate and are difficult to access for treatment. Building a healthy microbiota population with a high fiber organic diet, colonics and a targeted cleanse program are some of the best ways to remove these films/bio-shields and the colonies living in them. Probiotic supplementation, cultured and fermented foods, a low glycemic, alkalanising, gluten-free, fiber rich mostly raw plant based diet, all support a healthy gut.

Acid/Alkaline Balancing

Acids are defined as substances that release hydrogen ions when dissolved in water and the degree of acidity is measured by determining its PH (potential hydrogen). It is also possible to identify a food as acidic by analyzing mineral content as sulfur, chlorine, phosphorous, fluoride, iodine and silicon which are acidic, while calcium, sodium, magnesium, cobalt and copper are alkaline. Strong acids, because of their resistance to combining are much more difficult to neutralize and eliminate from the body than weak acids.

Strong acids come primarily from animal proteins, chiefly consisting of uric, sulfuric and phosphoric acids. Their elimination from the body requires significant neutralization, a task performed by the liver as well as the normal elimination work of the kidneys. Because the kidneys can only eliminate a fixed amount of strong acids on a daily basis, any excess is stored in the tissues. Weak acids (sometimes called volatile acids) are primarily of plant origin and are easily oxidized and eliminated by the lungs in the form of vapors and gasses.

"CAD, (Coronary Artery Disease) begins with progressive endothelial injury, inflammatory oxidative stress, and diminution of nitric oxide production, foam cell formation, and development of plaques that may rupture to cause a myocardial infarction (MI) or stroke. This cascade is set in motion in part by, and is exacerbated by, the western diet of added oils, dairy, meat, fowl, fish, sugary foods (sucrose, fructose, and drinks containing those, refined carbohydrates, fruit juices, syrups, and molasses) that injures or impairs endothelial function after each ingestion, making food choices a major, if not the major, cause of CAD."
-Caldwell Esselyn MD

~~~~

The body functions at its best when the Ph. of its internal biochemical environment is 7.39. Illness will accompany any incidence of acidosis (7.36-7 Ph.) and over half the population suffers from this condition. The slightest change in blood ph. is rapidly corrected by the body, restoring it to the ideal 7.39. If unable to do this task, physical and mental disorders appear quickly.

As the kidneys cannot eliminate more than a fixed amount each day, the body makes use of alkaline elements found in "less important" parts of the body, like the tissues of the internal organs. Problems occur when tissues are forced to relinquish their alkaline elements on a regular basis. Modern lifestyles and diet encourage such exploitation of the body's buffer system and this is the source of a host of troubles and diseases, as well as a general sense of malaise.

~~~~

"The acidity levels that literally are put into the body from a meat based diet, in and of themselves, cause the major impetus, or the major starting point for the cancers to start in the body. Now let's look at animal-based protein when it comes to acid. You get, for instance, eight parts of acid which we call RAL from eating animal-based proteins. Let's talk about what they are again so everyone's clear. We're not talking about red meat. I'm not talking about only red meat. I'm talking about fish consumption. I'm talking about chicken consumption. I'm talking about red meat. I'm talking about pork. I'm talking about dairy food." D. Clement

~~~~

Excess acidity can instigate problems with slower enzyme actions, eczema, red patches, hives, and itching from acids coming out through the skin and urinary tract as well as related infections (urethritis/cystitis) that commonly occur. Often there is an increased vulnerability to microbial or viral infection from the fragile state of tissues and hampered immune function. Acid caused demineralization can be most apparent with problems affecting the skeleton and teeth. A sustainably grown, whole foods, enzyme rich, plant based diet is a better option!

Enzymes and Raw Foods

What makes raw food so healthy is because it hasn't been cooked, it still has all of its nutrition and life-force intact. The naturally occurring enzymes in raw food allow for digestion, without tapping into the body's enzyme reserve. Then the body's enzymes are available for the process of detoxification, repair and healing. Rejuvenation rather than maintenance or degeneration happens with plant based, raw and living foods. We are able to grow younger and look better in the ongoing aging process of replacing our cells with better nourished more alive cells!

~~~~

"Many of the diseases for which modern medicine has no cure are the result of complex, extremely gradual changes at the cellular level. Those changes are a direct consequence of a lifelong diet made mostly of processed sugary, fatty foods. An intensive plant based diet program is the fastest and most effective way to rejuvenate the body at the cellular level, and to give it the raw materials it requires to rebuild itself and function more effectively."
-D. Sandoval, *The Green Foods Bible*, Purium Foods

~~~~

When integrating more raw foods many start to feel better physically, more calm, optimistic, more harmonious in thoughts and feelings and even needing less sleep. This is largely because cooking, besides destroying life force rich enzymes, destroys 60-70% of the vitamins, makes 50% of the protein unavailable, destroys much of the B12 and completely eliminates the phytonutrients so important for life force, energy and health.

Raw foods contain their full complement of nutrients and are abundant with the enzymes needed to turn food into energy the body can use. Plants have the magical ability to photosynthesize energy from the sun, that is then stored in their cells. With fresh raw food this life force (like electrical energy) can be assimilated to recharge us!

~~~~

"The trace elements, enzymes and cofactors present in raw, whole foods actually make the "nutrient" or antioxidant work! A whole food-based nutrient supplement can deliver nutritional punch because of improved bioavailability and synergy between the various nutrients. Vibrant health is based on choosing the world's healthiest foods, concentrated, not mega doses of isolated vitamins, minerals, and whatever other nutrients or phytochemicals all tossed in."
-D. Sandoval, Purium Health Foods

Healthy digestion and absorption is of paramount importance in order to assimilate nutrition from food. Chewing well, proper food combining, healthy intestinal flora and the right foods all play an important part. When what we eat is nutritionally compromised and enzyme deficient, cooked foods, the pancreas must try to compensate by adding digestive enzymes. Over time this weakens the pancreas and creates poor digestion and assimilation, a major part in diabetes onset. Raw foods often have higher water contents, thereby providing hydration, along with the regularity supporting richness of fiber. Below are some of the most common experiences of people exploring a raw food diet; (includes info from www.karenknowler.com)

- Feeling on the way to reaching ones highest health potential
- Feeling lighter in body, mind and soul
- Feeling more connected to self and the world
- Having more love and patience with others
- Feeling as if we can more easily know our life purpose and pursue it
- Falling in love with an unfolding new life
- Rejuvenating and reversing signs of aging
- Detoxifying the body naturally
- Strengthening the immune system
- Improved memory, sharper concentration

Explore the huge variety of extraordinary raw foods in the shopping list - Resources section. Next is a sampling of the wide variety of super healthy and delicious raw foods available:

- Fresh fruits (apples, pears, papaya, cherimoya, pineapple etc.)
- Vegetables (carrots, broccoli, cauliflower, sweet potatoes etc.)
- Salad vegetables (tomatoes, bell peppers, cucumbers etc.)
- Leafy green vegetables (kale, spinach, chard etc.)
- Herbs (basil, cilantro, parsley etc.)
- Wild greens (dandelion, nettle, purslane etc.)
- Nuts (macadamia, walnut, Brazil etc.)
- Dried fruits (dates, raisins, apricots, prunes etc.)
- Sprouted beans, pulses and legumes (adzuki, mung, lentil etc.)
- Sprouted grains (wheat, rye, barley etc.)
- Seeds (pumpkin, black-sesame, sunflower, hemp, chia etc.)
- Sprouted seeds (quinoa, buckwheat, flax etc.)
- Indoor greens (wheatgrass/kamut grass, sunflower greens, etc.)
- Sprouted vegetable seeds (broccoli, mustard, fenugreek etc.)
- Sea vegetables (dulse, wakame, kelp etc.)

- Algae's (chlorella, spirulina, Klamath lake blue-green algae etc.)
- Oils (coconut, olive, sesame, hemp, etc.)
- Strong spices (onion, garlic, cayenne pepper, etc.)
- Spices (turmeric, ginger, cumin, cinnamon nutmeg etc.)
- Flavorings and sweeteners (coconut nectar, lucuma, stevia etc.)
- Superfoods (aloe vera, cacao, goji berries, maca, etc.)
- Pre-packaged, prepared raw foods (nut butters, seed butters, flax crackers etc.)

~~~~

"As a researcher interested in finding out the truth about how the body could rejuvenate and heal itself, I have been truly blessed to have studied with and be inspired by some of the most respected personalities in the field of alternative medicine, including Ann Wigmore, the mother of wheatgrass therapies and the greatest proponent of living foods. She showed me that one person's selflessness and love for others could change the world. She was like Mother Theresa, helping people find dignity and hope, in their most desperate and needy times." -David Sandoval, The Green Foods Bible, Purium Foods

Plant Based, the Health, Environmental and Ethical Considerations

Over 20 years ago one of the most profound, wise, and comprehensive holistic health teachers I have ever known asked me a life changing question, "how do you expect to find peace and happiness when you are eating pain and suffering?" Being that I was brought up in Hawaii, where the family business was one of the biggest restaurant food supply companies, embracing veganism and cleansing, to connect with my true self, was a monumental shift.

After reading Ann Wigmores, *Recipes for Longer Life* and John Robbins book, *Diet for a New America*, I deepened my commitment to embracing a plant based diet and lifestyle. That choice then led me to my unknown, innate, skills as a vegan chef/caterer and passion for understanding holistic health. I also found a deeper commitment to living freedom and infinite possibilities through embracing major cleansing, emotional healing, and release of limiting beliefs, all supported by a vegan, compassionate, spiritually based, more connected and healthy life.

~~~~

"Spiritual vegetarianism is a spiritual practice that links us to the rest of nature and the rest of our own nature. Spiritual vegetarianism acknowledges the interconnectedness of all beings and enacts compassion towards them. It acts on the understanding that we express ourselves through relationships and that these relationships include the other animals. Spiritual vegetarianism is a living Ahimsa, the absence of violence." -Carol Adams, The Inner Art of Vegetarianism

Now years later, the relevance of that shift has become even more apparent, as my own, appropriate, personal, most response-able choice to corporate animal agriculture- factory farming, which is at the top of the list, as the most devastating cause of a long list of World problems, at very center, core of all problems and generating them. This industry has gone totally bezerk, attacking, and critically endangering our very life support systems, devastating the Worlds environments and people's health, while breeding shallowness and ignorance!

Peace and sustainability depends on ending the behavior and mentality of domination and exploitation. The animal food industry slaughters 70 million animals a day, in the US alone, that have been imprisoned, tortured, heavily drugged and subjected to unimaginable suffering both in their lives and in the slaughtering process. All the while generating massive health and environmental catastrophes with huge amounts of sewage waste, greenhouse gasses, forest decimation, GMO feed production, human starvation, loss of topsoil, ocean dead zones and massive overfishing and on and on.

~~~~

"While the worlds rich omnivores waste precious supplies of grains, petroleum, land and water feeding and eating fattened animals the world's poor have little grain to eat or clean water to drink and their chronic hunger, thirst and misery create conditions for war, terrorism and drug addiction which are extremely profitable industries as well. The richest fifth of the world's population gets obesity, heart disease and diabetes, also highly profitable for industry. The system spreads relentlessly and globally and while corporate and bank returns may be healthy, people, animals, and ecosystems throughout the world fall ill and are exploited and destroyed..." World peace Diet, Will Tuttle

~~~~

The ignorant mass consuming of these pain, suffering and toxin filled, environmentally destructive, substances, breeds shallowness and ignorance in meal rituals that disconnects us from our inner lives. As we treat animals so do we treat each other as we exploit humans and condone torture, female domination, rape, war, slavery, pharmaceutical drugging....

~~~~

"We sow seeds of not just cancer, obesity, diabetes, and heart disease with our violence toward animals, but also of drug abuse, family breakdown, war, hunger, slavery, and exploitation because this is precisely how we behave toward cows, chickens, fish, and other animals for food, by the hundreds of millions every day. We are killing over sixty billion mammals and birds for food annually, plus an estimated one to two trillion marine animals, as well as untold billions more

animals who are killed as collateral damage as their habitats are destroyed and pesticides ravage global ecosystems." -World peace Diet, Will Tuttle

~~~~

There are over 2,000 different types of drugs and hormones that are given to these animals (cows, chickens, pigs, turkeys, fish). As we consume them we get sick and are given more drugs, including powerful psychotropic ones for those that get affected by eating the hormones, suffering and terror of these animals. We receive what we give, if we want mercy we must give it.

~~~~

"Three quarters of the food we grow is fed to imprisoned animals for meat and dairy, while roughly a billion people are chronically hungry and starving. The scale of the industrial killing machine of animals for food is so vast, it is mentally incomprehensible. Inevitably, the violence and heart-hardening required by this killing machine boomerangs in countless ways."
-Dr Will Tuttle, www.Worldpeacediet.org

~~~~

Our greatest joy is found by cultivating our sensitivity, inner awareness, wisdom and intuition, then acting with compassion, and being of service in the world. The best thing most of us can do is extricate ourselves from this disempowering, merciless tragedy, becoming more sensitive to the interconnectedness of all life. As we wean ourselves from this culturally induced trance of the meat industry's barbaric factory farm killing of animals for food, we can maintain and improve our health- we can more easily answer the high call of awakening our potential and leave this planet a better place for us having been here.

~~~~

"The more we realize our true self, the more we feel a connection with all life."
-At Home in the Universe

~~~~

Then we can create a habitable planet where the children are healthy and where sanity, kindness, mercy, health, and freedom prevail for all beings. Choosing a plant based diet is the most leveraged contribution most of us can make towards world peace, sustainability, health and freedom. A vegan diet can open the door to, or significantly add to, a heart-centered way of life.

~~~~

"We are called, now, to make an effort to make the connections between our massive ongoing violence toward animals for food and the mentality that is required for that, and the violence we all experience in the war and inequity of our culture. As we awaken from the obsolete cultural program of eating foods

sourced from animals, and change our behavior, we will be finally capable of creating a culture of loving kindness, equality, respect, freedom, abundance, joy, and sustainability. It is a beckoning possibility and always available." -Will Tuttle

~~~~

"The Department of Agriculture's promotional poster used to list milk as the first group and meat as the second. Grains got a group and fruits and vegetables had to share a group. Because livestock products were assigned two of the four groups, menus developed under this plan were often loaded with fat and cholesterol. This is how an entire generation learned to eat and how they in turn raised their children.

The results are tragic. There are 4,000 heart attacks every day in this country. The traditional four food groups and the eating patterns they prescribed have led to cancer and heart disease in epidemic numbers, and they have killed more people than any other factor in America. More than automobile accidents, more than tobacco, more than all the wars of this country combined." -Neil Barnard

~~~~

"Studies in Campbell's laboratory and elsewhere have demonstrated that without animal proteins in the diet the initiation process of cancer development is often stalled. It appears that regardless of the level of exposure of the initiating carcinogen, many cancers may be unable to develop and progress without the presence of animal protein in the diet." –Lislie/Goldhammer, The Pleasure Trap

~~~~

"In addition to calories and nutrients to support growth, cow's milk increases hormones that directly stimulate the growth of the calf. The most powerful of these hormones is called insulin-like growth factor-1 (IGF-1). When cow's milk is fed to people, IGF-1 levels also increase. Studies funded by the dairy industry show a 10% increase in IGF-1 levels in adolescent girls from one pint daily and the same 10% increase for postmenopausal women from 3 servings per day of nonfat milk or 1% milk.[4,5] This rise in IGF-1 level is an important reason for the "bone-building" effects of cow's milk.

IGF-1 promotes undesirable growth too—like cancer growth and accelerated aging. IGF-1 is one of the most powerful promoters of cancer growth ever discovered for cancers of the breast, prostate, lung, and colon.[6] Overstimulation of growth by IGF-1 leads to premature aging too—and reducing IGF-1 levels is "anti-aging." John McDougal MD

~~~~

"Avoid all animal, fish, and dairy products, foods known to injure endothelial cells, as well as exogenous cholesterol and saturated fat. In avoiding exposure to the lecithin and carnitine contained in eggs, milk and dairy products, liver, red meat, poultry, shellfish and fish, participants in our study were unlikely to have intestinal flora capable of producing trimethylamine oxide (TMAO), a recently identified atherogenic compound (injures blood vessel wall flexibility through hampering nitrous oxide production) produced by the intestinal flora unique to omnivores that ingest animal products. (Vegans do not possess the detrimental bacterial)"
-Caldwell Esselyn M.D.

~~~~

"Everything is connected, the consumption of dairy products and eggs is linked with allergies, skin disorders, cancer, heart disease, stroke, diabetes, and a laundry list of other ailments; the agenda of products and procedures marketed by the medical industry to combat these unnecessary ailments, the enormous profits accumulated by the agribusiness, chemical, pharmaceutical and banking industries from our domination of female animals, the social inequity and injustice that this promotes, giving rise to elitism and further conflict, the environmental and human health effects of agricultural runoff, which is poisoning rivers, killing fish, contributing to human cancer and causing red tides that inflict respiratory disease, the lives lost in wars caused by spiraling demand for petroleum and by desperation as water rights go to rich agribusiness dairy and chicken operations funded by US banks in Third World countries, while poor people face chronic thirst and contaminated water (to start)." -World peace Diet, Will Tuttle

~~~~

"Our routine violence toward trillions of animals for meat, fish, dairy products, and eggs is the primary driving force behind not just the environmental devastation on our planet, but also behind the cultural, economic, psychological, and physical disease we experience as well. As individuals and as a culture, our ability to heal, transform, and evolve beyond this old defiling mentality, is tied to our food choices more than to anything else. To meditate for world peace, to pray for a better world, and to work for social justice and environmental protection while continuing to purchase the flesh, milk and eggs of horribly abused animals, exposes a disconnect that is so fundamental that it renders our efforts absurd, hypocritical, and doomed to certain failure!" -World peace Diet, Will Tuttle

~~~~

"Maybe we aren't on a one way road to oblivion; maybe we are standing at a crossroad, facing what may be the most important choice human beings have ever faced, a choice between two directions. In one direction is what we will have if we do nothing to alter our present course. By doing nothing, we are choosing a world of pollution and extinctions, of widening chasms and deepening despair, a

world where humanity moves farther from achieving its highest aspirations and closer to living its darkest fears." -John Robbins, The Food Revolution

~~~~

"If you live with fear for our future you are not alone. If you live with dreams for a better world you are not alone. On this path we work responsibly and joyfully to make our lives and our society's, into expressions of our love for ourselves, for each other and for the living earth. In this direction we honor our longing to give our children, and all children, a world with clean air and water, with blue skies and abundant wildlife, with a stable climate and a healthy environment. We all live now with both the pain and the possibility we carry in our hearts, both the despair and the hope that we may yet learn to live in harmony with our precious and endangered Earth." -John Robbins, The Food Revolution (2001)

~~~~

"Part of the problem is that the toxins used in industrial agriculture are highly profitable for the wealthy and privileged elite that dominate our cultural conversations through its power over the media, government and education. The military-industrial-meat-medical-media complex has and offers no incentive to reduce animal food consumption. Poisoning the earth with massive doses of toxic chemicals and petroleum based fertilizers is highly profitable for the petroleum and chemical industries. These toxins cause cancer which is highly profitable for to the chemical-pharmaceutical—medical complex."
-World peace Diet, Will Tuttle

~~~~

"With its immense financial resources and legendary influence at all levels of government, animal agribusiness receives billions of dollars in subsidies, price supports, income assistance, emergency assistance , commodity loans, direct payments, allotments, tax breaks, rail and feed subsidies, grazing privileges, the dairy export incentive program, and other governmental services every year. Without this aid the industry could never survive in its present form; the cheapest hamburger meat would cost at least $35/lb without taxpayer funded irrigation systems, subsidies, remediation allowances and countless other government handouts." World peace Diet, Will Tuttle

~~~~

"Saying yes to plant-based, organic, unprocessed foods of life, freedom, and radiant health, grown in organic gardens, orchards, and fields and reflecting respect for the Earth and all living beings can transform our world. Let's work to understand the nature of the insidious cultural indoctrination that is devastating our world, remove it from our minds and our food habits (that means going plant based), and help others do the same we are all in this together." -Will Tuttle

Sustainability and a Healthy Soil-Food-Web

By "sustainable" it's meant that every year the "soil food web" will improve in health and productivity and every year fewer inputs are needed (fertilizer, pesticides, herbicides, water and energy) for greater, more profitable and healthier production."In a healthy soil with good organic matter and a healthy biology, a "soil-food-web" is created.

Plants exude simple sugars, proteins and carbohydrates in hundreds of different forms which then trigger responses from the soil biology. The bacteria, protozoa, beneficial nematodes and fungi respond to these triggers to provide the plants with nutrition and to protect the plants from disease. The biology accesses and holds water and contains plant nutrients within their own bodies and their own systems (in non-leachable forms) and "trades" them with the plants for mutual benefit.

Fungi have the ability to "wick" water and nutrients from many meters below the soil surface to the plant roots (reduce water needs by more than 30%). Funji also, along with Bacteria, have the ability to produce antibiotics to combat plant pathogens, and also to store vast amounts of nitrogen, that are made available to the plants through the actions of a healthy soil-food-web. Both beneficial fungi and beneficial bacteria successfully fight plant disease by occupying the sites on leaf and root surfaces where pathogens would otherwise attack.

Nutrients in the soil are in the proper forms for the plant to take-up. It is one of the functions of a healthy food-web to hold nutrients in non-leachable forms so they remain in soil, until the plant requires the nutrients. When the biology is functioning properly the soil "biome" is improved so water demand is reduced, the need for fertilizers is reduced, and plant production is increased.

~~~~

"Compared to large-scale industrial farms, small scale agro-ecological farms not only use fewer fossil fuel-based fertilizer inputs and emit less GHGs, including methane, nitrous oxide and carbon dioxide (CO_2), but they also have the potential to actually reverse climate change by sequestering CO_2 from the air into the soil year after year. According to the Rodale Institute, small-scale farmers could sequester more than 100% of current annual CO_2 emissions with a switch to widely available, safe and inexpensive agro-ecological management practices that emphasize diversity, traditional knowledge, agroforestry, landscape complexity, and water and soil management techniques, including cover cropping, composting and water harvesting. Importantly, agro-ecology can not only sequester upwards of 7,000 pounds of CO_2 per acre per year, but it can actually boost crop yields."- Fairworldproject.org (newsletter issue 10)

Sustainability by western definition means living in a way that allows our biological systems to remain diverse and productive indefinitely. According to UCLA.edu "Sustainability is most often defined as meeting the needs of the present without compromising the ability of future generations to meet theirs." Sustainability has 3 main pillars, one is economic or profit, two environmental or planet, three social or people. Each of these aspects can either contribute or detract from the goal of establishing human-ecosystem equilibrium.

Clean water, clean air, and balanced ecosystems are critical factors in the overall cost-benefit equation of any product or process. Presently most people are motivated by "me" rather than "we." This self-centered mindset is destroying our planet. Resources are being depleted at an alarming rate, and the future of the planet looks increasingly bleak.

"As overwhelming as it may seem, it is important not to lose sight of what it could look like in a world where harmony and respect for one another prevail. Imagine everyone on the planet worked together to care for the resources, and shared them so no one went without adequate food, water, or shelter

Imagine there are no separate countries and instead, there is a global consciousness of "one world" where unity, harmony and peace prevail. In this alternate world, scientists focus on discovering new renewable energy and life giving solutions to health concerns. The economy is based on helping people rather than hurting people. Animals and plants are revered and the human population feels part of the life cycle rather than the dominator of it.

Unlike planet Earth now, where war, poverty, and cruelty to humanity the animals and the environment prevail, this new world is peaceful, abundant and conscious of the underlying interconnectedness of all beings. There is a profound understanding if you hurt one, you hurt all. Fear and greed are not the driving forces, and instead. Life is honored and united."
Liah Howard- Summer 2017 Living Aloha magazine

GMO's, Now We Know

"No one has the right to play genetic roulette with the entire genetic integrity of life on this planet!" -Genetic Roulette Documentary (GAIAM.TV)

~~~~

Eating GMOs allows the consumption of foods soaked in herbicides. Animals eating GMO foods are shown to have much higher rates of cancer and other diseases. Since the introduction of GMOs kids allergies to food has increased dramatically (See Allergy Kids on GAIAM.TV). It has become obvious that there are absolutely no benefits to GMO and that it is one of the most glaring symbols of a completely unsound and destructive, greed based food production practice.

Americans get sick more often than Europeans and other industrialized countries. The top 3 chronic illnesses have doubled infant mortality rates increased and life-span years are plunging. This is not normal and there are reasons for this illness epidemic! The biggest change affecting people has been the introduction of GMOs and subsequent mass production of BGH, Bovine Growth Hormone, in milk. This along with GMO crops, especially BT corn and Roundup Ready Soy being produced on over 100 million acres in the US.

In both herbicide tolerant and pesticide producing gene insertion, swapping genes and cloning makes hundreds-of-thousands of mutations up and down the DNA. When the electromagnetic sensors of the immune system come across these foreign gene sequence signatures it responds with an inflammatory reaction attack. The incidence of gut inflammation, ulcerative colitis, and numerous gut disorders have risen since 1996, as have allergies, autoimmune diseases, diabetes and heart disease. People and farm animals have been consuming these *bad science foods* for almost 20 years and the results in polluted earth and epidemics of ill health are beyond extreme.

Allergies to food have skyrocketed in recent years and with the prescribing of a non GMO, organic diet, symptoms are often alleviated. In rats, pigs and cattle consuming GMO feed, inflamed, irritated stomachs are common. These same symptoms are strikingly similar to the gut inflammation often prevalent in Autistic Spectrum Disease. When GMO is taken out of the animals' diet there is an obvious positive behavioral change and relief from digestive ailments.

When Roundup herbicide is used the active ingredient Glyphosate turns off photosynthesis and blocks plant nutrient uptake. This not only causes non-Roundup ready plants to starve, it lowers the available nutrients in plants treated with roundup making them weak and sick. Animals fed these crops become nutrient deficient and these animals and plants, when used for human consumption make people weak and sick. Glyphosate has a detrimental effect on gut bacteria, in humans as well. Time and time again when animal farms switch from GMO feed, disease rates plummet, as do birth defects and stomach related illnesses, while conception rates, as well as positive behavior, increase.

The US has had a huge increase in childhood disease, to the point where we have the highest rates of Asthma, Autism, ADHD, Allergies and Cancer and where 1 in 3 kids has one of these illnesses. Many overseas countries that banned GMO and BGH have much lower rates, many with virtually no Autism at all. In 27 countries GMO is not allowed and in 60 others it must be labeled.

Overseas, the same companies sell the same labeled products, but don't have artificial dies, GMOs etc. ingredients because of consumer demand and government regulation.

Many consumers are not aware of the dangers of the science involved and the biotech industry's control and involvement in the highest levels of the USDA and FDA. Many employees of the biotech industry have positions in government regulatory bodies. The Biotech's master plan is to eliminate all natural seed worldwide, replace it with GMO seed and have a huge market for their chemicals. People that have spoken up are attacked, fired from jobs and discredited. Scientists, professors, researchers all face funding cancellations, shredded reputations and various threats. Recently released memos from the FDA, that were totally ignored, show an overwhelming consensus, even from their own GMO scientists, warning of the health dangers of this science.

.

Kids in the US today are often referred to as the RX generation, ideal for fitting a reoccurring revenue model of a continually sick child on diabetic or allergy medicine for the rest of their life. A sick cradle to grave business model for pharmaceutical companies.

Many parents are waking up, starting to become educated and take action as food allergies escalate in numbers and life threatening strength. Pediatric Cancer is now the fastest growing disease in the US and new Pediatric hospitals can hardly be built fast enough to handle the huge increases in patients. This combined with serious gut illnesses, diabetes etc. are threatening to buckle the health care system.

Mental Health, the Starving Brain and Pharmaceutical Madness

For many patients, psychiatric symptoms are often warning signs of underlying issues, including nutritional deficiencies and toxin exposures that impact physical health as well. Failure to look for and detect a possible underlying medical cause, or contributing factors, often unnecessarily prevents the alleviation of, extends or deepens the psychosis and underlying problem of the patient.

While modern medicine, used judiciously, can be valuable and lifesaving at times the general practice of "managing symptoms" all too often ends up making things worse. Masking signs of other unhealthful conditions invariably leads to increased ill health. It has become obvious much of the mental health diagnostics and resulting pharmaceutical prescriptions are all too often, clearly inaccurate. It is estimated that there are 100 million people worldwide and 8 million American children on these mostly mis-prescribed medications! Thank goodness for the

Complimentary Alternative Medicine Doctors looking at the whole picture and using proven nutritional formulas, cleansing protocols and lifestyle changes to remedy this mistaken situation.

~~~~

"When we have about half the population in North America alone on some level of pharmaceutical drug, that's pretty impressive and pretty frightening at the same point how they were able to achieve such a thing. In the United States we take double the amount of pharmaceutical drugs than any other nation in the world. That's a frightening proposition. When they've convinced us we have disorders we really don't have and they're putting drugs out as was pointed out earlier on about the standards for research, drugs on the market that have these major side effects." -Dr. Brian Clement

~~~~

I was somewhat unaware of the enormity of this situation and the severity of withdrawal from these drugs until a recent visit to New Zealand. While there we met up with some longtime friends who are experienced health coaches. At the time we also met with a midwife whom they were helping withdraw from some prescription medications she had been given for depression. This depression was really caused by adrenal fatigue from, staying up late and working hard at the hospital. She was prescribed drugs that were so addictive, if she missed even one dose, her whole body would go into racking pain.

Our friends had been coaching her for close to a year, giving her aloevera, high mineral, sea-weed supplements and having her take a few less of the pharmaceuticals grains (titrate) each day until she was finally able to discontinue. I have since come to know the sad reality and toll of harmful pharmaceutical based prescriptions when dealing with psychiatric imbalances, symptoms, and syndrome diagnosis. Not only do people often get worse, many suicides, mass murders and other violent actions are attributed to the non-judicious prescribing of these drugs.

Pharmaceutical companies are in the business of making money and disease maintenance, not in the business of curing people, for that would be bad business. Even though it's been shown healing the gut, heavy metal chelation, detoxification, nutrition, diet, lifestyle enhancement and exercise work much more effectively to maintain health and with much less cost, the pharmaceutical companies continue to earn 5 to 6 times more money than any other fortune 500 companies. The term "we are being Pharmed" is becoming all to true!

We have become a human commodity, cash cows, taking toxic substances that are riddled with misinformation about consequences and side effects. Most of it is a virus-like, parasitic industry, (once again we are truly grateful for the times of acute situations when pharmaceuticals are lifesaving) run amuck and thankfully we are at a crossroads to take our power back and have accountability for actions and for the many defective products and falsification of safety studies!

~~~~

"If we accept an inflammatory model of mental illness as having the strongest prospects for guiding preventive medicine interventions and non-toxic, reparative treatment approaches, then we must look at underlying drivers of inflammation.

Immune activating and inflammatory proteins, such as those found in wheat and dairy products, may be critical triggers to consider. One of the mostly highly processed foods in our diet - wheat – is almost exclusively rendered as high-glycemic flour, prepared with sugar, and often genetically modified vegetable oils which are oxidized (rancid). Dairy is homogenized and pasteurized, creating a dead, high-sugar liquid with distorted fats, denatured proteins and unabsorbable or thoroughly destroyed vitamins." -Kelly Brogan MD

~~~~

Thank goodness for the more enlightened pioneer physicians and health professionals who use functional, complementary and alternative medicine treatments (CAM). These are medical doctors, actually working as integrative practitioners, who look at the whole person, producing real and improved results of true recovery and wellness.

~~~~

"As a society, we can begin to think about protecting the microbiome by demedicalizing birth and infant nutrition, and as individuals, by avoiding antibiotics, NSAIDs, processed grains, genetically modified and non-organic food. Promising interventions for depression from a gut-brain perspective include probiotics, fermented foods as part of a high natural fat diet, and relaxation response for optimal digestion, anti-inflammatory and insulin sensitizing effects." -Kelly Brogan MD

~~~~

The CAM approach offers the practitioner many more options for progressively working towards a state of wellness for the client. Given the widespread positive results and rapid advance of research into CAM treatments, the orthodox paradigm is starting to shift. CAM looks at illness in a more holistic way:

1. Treat the whole person, mind, body, spirit, and environment.
2. Look for the deepest root problems, beneath the symptoms, which include using the best testing methods science has to offer.

3. Apply a continuum of treatments, always beginning with the safest, most natural, and most benign.

In some more up-to-date medical circles, the physician who ignores CAM may now be considered the less learned. A wise, truly caring physician, on the lookout for such risk factors, could actually save a patient years or even a lifetime of misdiagnosis, and add years of more healthful living rather than continued decline! Many drugs, particularly in combination, add more toxic substances to an already impaired body, producing more psychiatric symptoms, while CAM treatments work with the body chemistry.

Compared to drug therapy, natural treatments offer safer, more user friendly solutions, with far fewer and less harmful side effects. As studies now show, there is a real place for nutritional treatments in mental health treatment. When nutritional deficiencies are alleviated and the starving brain is fed people are then more able to take the next step of getting off these drugs. Second stage healing can then be addressed.

It has been unequivocally proven in court, in science and in practice by one amazing nutritional supplement that much of mental illness is first rooted and caused by absorption issues, leading to micronutrient deficiency. The potentised, balanced, bio available vitamin, mineral, amino acid formula, originally known as True Hope, is truly a miracle. Its subsequent testing by multiple universities, including by the head of Psychiatry at Harvard Medical School, and many peer reviewed and medical journal published studies, make it the most scientifically tested natural nutritional supplement in the world.

The details of the amazing story of Autumn Stringhams recovery from extreme psychological illness through her father's unrelenting research, determination and prayers can be found in her book, A Promise of Hope. This book details Autumn's miraculous recovery and the resulting development of the Q96 multivitamin mineral supplement.

Q96 is the most proven and successful formulation to facilitate the safe tapering off and discontinued need or use of SSRIs, anti-depressants, Bi-polar, schizophrenia etc. drugs and aid in full recovery. Q96 proves unequivocally that most mental illness is rooted in brain malnourishment. It even has the only support center of its kind, Micronutrient Research, having over 10 years of knowledge gained and over 90,000 people helped to safely withdraw from their pharmaceutical drug prescriptions.

It is now widely recognized that diet plays a significant role in mental wellbeing and overall health. The simple logic behind the consumption of healthy whole foods and the therapeutic use of natures, nutrient dense, concentrated superfoods has become clear. Food allergies can also show up with psychiatric symptoms, such as depression and anxiety, caused by food additives that many individuals are sensitive to. An excess of junk food can negatively affect mood and behavior, sometimes to a pathological level.

Toxic exposures of many kinds can dramatically influence mood, perception, and actions. Pesticides, mercury, gases, pollutants, lead, and even mycotoxins (microbial excretions) are suspects as mood changers. Safely getting off these drugs, supplying proper exercise and nutrition, then shifting the effects of ones diet from a heavily sugared, processed, and chemical loaded one, to a plant based, GMO free, gluten and casein free, rich in organic fruits-vegetables, whole grains, beans, seeds etc. diet is proven to have a dramatic impact on physical and mental health.

~~~~

"Are we to be blind sheep, led to the slaughter following the way of the World, eating man made, nutrient starved and depleted foods?" –Robyn Boyd

~~~~

With allergies increasing, Electro Magnetic Frequencies (EMFs) and toxic exposures on the rise in our increasingly industrialized world, psychiatric symptoms from these environmental causes are also becoming more prominent. Many typical psychiatric complaints such as anxiety, depression, even schizophrenia are frequently related to biochemical imbalances. These can range from low blood sugar-hyperglycemia, viral and fungal infections, hormonal imbalance, allergies and toxic overload, to deficiencies of specific nutrients. CAM physicians diagnose conditions with the appropriate laboratory tests that give a scientific basis for treatment.

This Functional or Integrative medicine then addresses the interactive systems of the whole person. The patient is evaluated in a variety of ways and supplied with specific health prescriptions for supplements, foods, exercise, natural hormones, and mind body techniques.

One situation that is often worked with is impaired methylation. (See Happy Healthy Hormones in following chapter). Methyl groups include B vitamins among others that play a crucial role in body systems, including hormone balance and liver function. Methylation de-activates noradrenalin, for example, a neurotransmitter associated with cortisol and the stress response. Methylation acts on dopamine, norepinephrine and serotonin to impact, among other things, mood, memory, concentration and sleep.

.

For the methylation cycle to work properly, the correct substrates, or materials, must be available. Nutrients involved in this activity include folic acid, B6, B12 and SAM-e. Other nutritional factors found to influence mood and brain functions are; essential fatty acid deficiency, blood sugar imbalance and brain inflammation due to food allergy's (i.e. gluten, casein), heavy metals, yeast etc.

A natural approach to Mental Health can include;

- Bio-available supplementation with amino acids, nutrient dense, concentrated superfoods, minerals, herbs, anti-oxidants and more to restore normal brain functions and immune response.
- Added supplementation with enzymes, essential fatty acids, algae's.
- As little medication as needed, avoiding an abrupt withdrawal from current medications.
- Dietary changes to reduce or eliminate junk foods, incorporate healthy foods, and remove offending foods, particularly chemicalized and allergy producing GMO and non-organic ones.
- Taking steps for repopulating beneficial bacteria in the gut microbiota and to heal any "leaky gut" issues.
- Exercise recommendations as needed.
- Hormonal treatments including herbal formulas.
- Detoxification, heavy metal chelation, and other natural or safe approaches to full recovery.
- Relaxation techniques including breathwork, yoga and meditation.
- Lifestyle changes including: living arrangements, job situation, marital counseling, and removing sources of stress.

~~~~

"Psychiatric diagnoses appear to be based on dubious science. Of the 297 mental disorders (now closer to 400) contained with the Diagnostic and Statistical Manual of Mental Disorders, none can be objectively measured by pathological tests. Mental illness symptoms within this manual are arbitrarily assigned by a subjective voting system in a psychiatric panel. It is estimated that 100 million people globally use psychotropic drugs. The Marketing of Madness film exposes the real insanity in our psychiatric 'health care' system: profit-driven drug marketing at the expense of human rights. This film plunges into an industry corrupted by corporate greed and delivers a shocking warning from courageous experts who value public health over dollar." -Marketing of Madness, film trailer

~~~~

Autism, the Gut Connection, and Brain Malnourishment

Autism Spectrum Disease and for that matter, ADHD, Asperger's and many mental health situations involve the interplay of gastrointestinal challenges and immune dysregulations leading to neurological impairment ramifications. Autism Spectrum Disease and many associated symptoms/illnesses have underlying malabsorption, maldigestion and other weakening mechanisms leading to malnourishment, a starving brain and improper neuronal function. Gastrointestinal inflammation and its underlying causes contribute to a cascade of other difficulties that constitute a major part of the disease process in many ASD children.

The interference in the flow of nutrients can impair consciousness, cognition, speech and behavior. Commonly, leaky gut allows undigested gluten and casein (soy also) proteins into the bloodstream forming drug like substances called opioids. These drug like proteins interfere with motivation, emotions, perceptions, response, normal brain development, while over stimulating nerve synapses and blocking normal signal transmissions to the brain. Gastrointestinal pathology leads to nutritional deficiencies, all of which can be treated!

~~~~

"Understanding that the gut and brain are connected helps explain why Autism, ADHD and overall health are improved through a diet that supports digestion, GI health and biochemistry. GI health and Biochemistry are partners. Biochemistry involves cellular processes that require energy, nutrients and enzymes to function and proper digestion is required to obtain and absorb the nutrients needed for these processes. Biochemistry can go awry if there are insufficient nutrients, an inability to digest and absorb nutrients, a limitation on a particular nutrient, or inability to convert a nutrient to the active and usable form. Attention to diet is crucial." -Julie Matthews, Nourishing Hope for Autism

~~~~

The liver secretes bile into the intestine during digestion which lubricates intestinal walls. Bile regulates the level of friendly bacteria, destroys unwanted and dangerous organisms, and stimulates peristaltic action to move fecal matter out of body. Bile, along with digestive fluid from the pancreas acts upon fats, protein, and starches transforming them into useful substances. Also the liver's job is to keep the bloodstream free of damaging poisons.

When the liver is not able to neutralize toxic substances because it is overworked, weak and congested from constipation, overeating/obesity, chemicalised food, Candida overgrowth etc. toxic bile is secreted. This creates inflamed tissue throughout the small intestine and is one of the leading causes of leaky gut syndrome and increased Candida overgrowth. Candida overgrowth due to antibiotic use, toxic mercury build up, and allergies to chemicalised, highly processed, and GMO foods increases this challenging picture.

Candida related complex can show up as many symptoms like Candida overgrowth commonly being found with Chronic Fatigue, Cancer, Aids, Epstein bar, Bronchitis, Pneumonia, and with increased immune system deficiencies. The fungus can quickly spread into the blood stream and begin creating colonies of yeast in and on every organ; (a systemic infection). As yeast multiplies it produces toxic waste products that circulate, poisoning and weakening the immune and endocrine system and polluting the brains neuronal function.

Another major factor in gut health and brain neurology is exposure to toxic metals. Mercury and other heavy metals can adversely affect the gastrointestinal, immune, nervous and endocrine systems. These toxins alter cellular function and numerous metabolic processes in the body, including those related to central and peripheral nervous systems. Lifelong disabilities are linked to toxic exposures of lead, mercury, other heavy metals and pesticides prevalent in the environment, often with exposure during early childhood or even before birth.

Heavy metals are bio-accumulative-they can chemically bond to molecules in mammalian bodies and be passed up the food chain to humans. Ingested mercury can be passed to the fetus in the womb of pregnant mothers from mercury amalgams when she chews and particularly when she has had dental work while pregnant. It's been shown how mercury poisoning causes speech and hearing deficits, sensory disturbances, aversion to touch and cognitive and behavioral impairments. These same impairments are present in ASD.

Many ASD children show major improvement in response to physician supervised heavy metal chelation, when combined with gut healing and nutritional support! Some researchers and physicians have postulated that when a particularly susceptible child suffers an environmental "insult" such as exposure to mercury, or even to the weakened viruses in vaccines, the child's immune system reacts. It not only attacks the actual antigens but also the look alike antigens that are actually molecular structures within the child's brain. When the immune system attacks the body's own myelin nerve protecting sheaths, short circuits can occur, with corresponding nerve axions ceasing to function properly.

Mercury poisoning leads to cognitive social deficits, loss of speech, poor concentration, word comprehension difficulties, sleep difficulties, (often exacerbated by heartburn and digestive pain issues), self-injurious behavior, agitation, unprovoked crying, and staring spells. Many children with mercury toxicity, or those having had early rounds of antibiotics, have reoccurring Otitis

Media (ear) infections. In most affected individuals the infections are not the primary cause of Autism or ADHD, they may be a first step, because Otitis Media is generally presumed to have an infectious bacterial origin and then generally treated with multiple antibiotics.

~~~~

"But we don't have to look at an injection and point our finger to one area. We just have to look at the environment. We look at everything from what we eat. And many of the pesticides, fungicides and herbicides are riddled with heavy metals. We look at the water we drink. We look at the air we breathe, we look at pharmaceutical drugs, riddled with heavy metals and chemicals. We look at the clothing we wear, riddled with heavy metals. And right down the list of things: the environment, the house you're living in, how about the rug in your home. And all of these add up to a very toxic environment that we live in. And the problem is that this is invisible to us." -Brian Clement

~~~~

Almost all ASD children have long standing vitamin and mineral deficiencies with subnormal uptake. Many children begin to improve when they begin a strong nutrient program, even before heavy metal detoxification has begun. Welcome nutrition helps the child's own immune and detoxification system to function better. It has become understood that mercury impairs the immune system, interferes with certain enzyme systems and allows yeast colonizing bacteria and even some viruses to get a firm hold on gut tissue.

Along with certain food hyper-sensitivities it interferes with nutrient transport across intestinal membranes and makes it chronically difficult for a child to receive adequate brain nourishment. Inadequate availability of nutrients can also reduce immunity and make it difficult to heal the opportunistic infections so common in ASD children. Many ASD children have entered into a vicious cycle of intestinal pathology, suboptimal nutrition, weakened immunity, impaired detoxification with subsequent accumulation of toxic metals. Such children are extremely vulnerable and susceptible to further injections of live viruses.

Autism is a complex syndrome involving genetic predisposition, the digestive and immune system, toxin laden food, a leaky gut, viral, fungal, and other pathogen invasions and an inability to detoxify poisons from heavy metals and pesticides. There are now many integrative physicians and many studies showing how to find real help in solving ASD situations. Check www.starvingbrains.com and www.Nourishinghope.com for excellent Autism treatment support.

First steps are to integrate a healthy diet, including eliminating GMOs, gluten, casein, soy, and corn and supplementing with concentrated, bio-available superfoods. Also important is healing the gut with glutamine, aloe vera juice, digestive enzymes, probiotics and cultured vegetables.

Supplementing with antivirals like oregano oil, olive leaf extract, grape seed extract, while detoxing the liver with milk thistle and other supplements can help. Having heavy metal chelation or exploring a zeolite, fulvic mineral combo as outlined in the *Longevity Source cleanse* can make a huge difference! With major health challenges, seeking professionally administered heavy metal chelation and overall support is recommended.

<center>~~~~</center>

"Considering the combination of factors that appear to contribute to Autism, the helpful effects of chlorella for autistic children are unsurprising. It aids in mercury detoxification, it contains high concentrations of anti-oxidants, and is packed with vitamins and minerals in highly bio-available forms. This makes it ideal for filling in nutritional gaps commonly found in the diets of autistic children."
-David Sandoval, The Green Foods Bible

Detoxification

The medical statistics of illness, mortality and suffering are beyond crisis! There is an epidemic of mostly unnecessary and avoidable, multiple degenerative conditions sweeping the US. Specific real causes, for virtually all health problems, are readily discernible and by taking responsibility for one's own healthcare we become empowered to create superior health and longevity rather than experiencing the anguish and suffering of becoming more medical statistics!

When it comes to accidents, injuries, physical therapy, emergencies and some corrective surgeries, medical services are invaluable, as I can well attest! A few times in emergency situations I have been extremely grateful for modern medical care and have found many genuinely caring doctors and staff! For many reasons though, including continued corporate profits, the medical profession treats diseases as things you get, with symptoms that are best pharmaceutically/ chemically suppressed.

Illness is processes we develop due mostly to factors/choices under our control. At this point, to be free of illness a "pound" of prevention could be worth one's life! Sad but true, if we wait till we become dangerously toxic, and our health becomes overly compromised, illness often becomes biologically less probable to reverse, with lethal results. It's a very humbling and sobering experience to personally attend a detox and healing center such as Optimum Health Institute or Hippocrates and closely share the physical, emotional, and mental cleansing/

re-education process with individuals who are struggling to overcome conditions labeled "terminal."

Western diet has become increasingly rich in meats, poultry, saturated fats, GMOs, refined chemicalized processed foods, salt, sugar, and alcohol. The overgenerous intake of animal fats has burdened the cardiovascular systems with cholesterol, kidneys with protein, and livers with animal hormones and drugs. Processed foods accounts for more than half of most Americans diet, are loaded with refined sugars, preservatives, artificial and chemically altered ingredients (anti-nutrients).

~~~~

"The saddest things I work with today are the young, young, young people coming to us with catastrophic stage 4 cancers and other diseases. Diabetes, two out of three people contracting diabetes today are youngsters below 16. I have a close friend, and she left nursing. She was one of my favorite people in medicine because this woman cared. She worked in the ER for her whole career, and recently left. And I said, "Why did you leave? You loved it so much". She said, "I couldn't take another 20-year-old coming in with a heart attack and dying in front of me in the emergency room". And I said, "It's that common? She said, "Yes." -Brian Clement, Hippocrates Institute

~~~~

Almost all disease begins by the accumulation of toxins in the body and living in a toxic environment. Over ninety percent of all the toxins that are taken in enter through the intestinal lining. Even toxins from the air we breathe pass through the intestines. These toxins become caught in the mucous linings of the mouth or nasal passages and then drain into the stomach, making their way into the intestines. The intestinal lining is often exposed to millions of toxins daily!

~~~~

"Many experts in the medical community believe that true health starts in the gut. Digestive issues can affect the body as a whole, contributing to everything from allergies and acne to IBS, liver disease, mood swings and even cancer. Your gut also shields your immune system, so when it's compromised, you're more vulnerable to becoming sick. Dietary imbalances (too much sugar, processed foods, overeating), medication use, mineral deficiencies and even stress can also change the balance of bacteria in your digestive tract, leaving you susceptible to a host of different health conditions." -Dr. Sarah Gottfried, The Hormone Cure

~~~~

A stressful schedule can also lead people to eat on the run. Most fast food diets include large portions of meat, fat, and sugar, and very little fresh vegetables, whole grains, and water. This type of low fiber diet can lead to stress, a backed-up colon and diverticulitis. Stressed individuals also skip meals or eat on the go. Just as a regular eating schedule leads to regular bowel movements inconsistent or rushed meals can likewise lead to problems in the gut and constipation.

Toxic intestines are simply not able to function properly because they are inhibited by layers of accumulated toxins, which become impacted waste material. This creates a narrowed passageway leading to constipation and other bowel problems. Constipation makes having regular bowel movements difficult and leads to further impaction. If toxins are not eliminated from the intestines on a regular basis, they leach back into the bloodstream through what is called "leaky gut syndrome" where they can ultimately cause disease.

These toxins make their way into the bloodstream, subsequently causing blood toxemia or congestive toxicosis, overworking the liver, and then infiltrating every type of tissue. In tissue they cause degenerative diseases and emotional distress throughout the body. These chemicals disrupt sensitive biochemical and hormonal balances by altering the electrical signals in the water within blood and living cells, thus causing depression, mood disorders, and other disturbances.

Candida overgrowth easily occurs and the excessive Candida also robs the body of essential nutrients by consuming starches and sugars in the digestive tract. As Candida consumes food, like any other living organism, it also produces waste. This waste is toxic to the human body and can cause a wide range of symptoms, frequently confused with other disorders. If undigested food remains in the body too long, proteins putrefy (producing toxic ammonia, hydrogen sulfide and other toxins), carbohydrates ferment (producing ethyl alcohol or lactic acid), and fats turn rancid (creating highly reactive toxic molecules which destroy nutrients and vitamins). This changes the compounds in the food so they become harmful instead of beneficial. This rotten food collects inside the colon, making regular bowel movements increasingly difficult.

It is generally accepted that bowel movement frequency can range from three per day to three per week, but some people have just two or less per week. The fermentation, putrefaction, rancidity, and sheer amount of toxins leaking into the bloodstream from a polluted colon that produces only two or three bowel movements a week is unimaginable. A person with a healthy elimination system should have two, three or four well formed, effortless, low odor, bowel movements daily. This means disease starts in the digestive tract and health begins in the digestive track. Skillful living starts with having a clean body, and a home and work environment that are free from toxic chemicals and disease causing agents.

~~~~

"With lifestyle and stress serving as the number one contributors to disease and pathology in our current world, Vitality understands the urgency of combating and thoroughly addressing these concerns. Our model is based on the premise that basic diet, nutrition, supplements, exercise, sleep habits, stress management, and mindset are critical components of proper health. Our goal is to maintain balance and preserve health by treating all necessary aspects of a person's life."
-Pedram Shojai, Vitality movie

~~~~

The pharmaceutical industry, government-funded medical research, and huge numbers of around-the-clock medical staff would be unnecessary, if people discovered and practiced, the way to achieve optimal health was to keep their intestines, liver, body, and living environment clean. This would, though, cause the loss of hundreds of billions of dollars in annual health care revenue through the "health care" industry's persistent denial of preventative care.

Regaining health is often as easy as cleansing our bodies regularly and slowly changing the environments in which we live and work, then as a society, we wouldn't need or be dependent upon prescription drugs or worrying about a decaying environment.

This concept doesn't match with the pharmaceutical profit driven incentives of addressing only symptoms instead of root causes of disease! It's stupefying to consider how many Americans are taking drugs they don't really need instead of addressing the underlying cause of their health problems. Obviously, both the medical establishment and the pharmaceutical industry are the only ones benefiting from this inconsistency and even many doctors are becoming disillusioned.

~~~~

"[M]any of our most crippling conditions could be greatly reduced, if not completely eradicated, simply by eating what they call a "whole foods plant based diet." This means consuming foods that come mainly from whole minimally refined plants, such as fruits, vegetables, grains, and legumes. It also means avoiding animal based foods, such as meat, dairy, and eggs. As well as processed foods like bleached flours, refined sugars, and oil." -John Robbins

~~~~

To become aware of the many toxin sources and take steps to eliminate them is to take a major step towards responsibility for one's own health!

Toxins- Some of the main physical (and mental) illness causing factors:

White flour, GMO processed soy/corn, pesticides, genetically modified foods, MSG, hydrogenated oils, fast and fried foods, boxed, canned, processed foods
Pasteurized milk, soft drinks, diet colas, "energy" (highly caffeinated) drinks
High fructose corn syrup (GMO), irradiated foods
Chemically poisoned and heavy metal contaminated fish
Fillers, binders, artificial colorings
Prescription drugs, overused antibiotics, animal antibiotics in food
Coffee, alcohol, refined sugars, artificial sweeteners, Aspartame
Tap water toxins include, arsenic, fluoride, chlorine, prescription drug residues, pesticides, Bisphenol-A (toxin used in making plastic water bottles), C8 (the chemical used to make Teflon®.
Bacteria, yeast, fungus, worms, amoebas, viruses, molds, mildew, Candida, parasites and the poisonous micotoxins produced by all the above.
Fallates/plasticizers in plastic water bottles that become Endocrine system disrupting Xenoestrogens- herbicides, pesticides
Household cleaners, bug sprays. birth control pills, other hormone disruptors.
Benzene, paint fumes, synthetic chemicals, liver toxic glues
Body "care" products, sunscreens, deodorants, perfumes etc.
Ionizing radiation, CAT scans, x rays, microwave cooking, power lines, cell phones, computers, household appliances, fluorescent lighting, hair dryers,
Heavy metals from cookware, mercury dental fillings, vaccines, cosmetics, aluminum cans, commercial food, light bulbs, many non-organic commercial herbal supplements, toothpaste, household and automobile paints, etc.
.

Other Health Challengers:

Stress induced high cortisol levels
Gluten and other food allergies
Depressed thyroid from gluten allergy's, heavy metals, toxins
Lack of strong pancreatic enzymes from too much cooked and processed food.
Acidic body PH (sugar, meat, coffee, chemical food, lack of exercise, (cancer only grows in an acidic environment).
Fibrin, bad calcium, and other plaque like materials causing stagnation and harboring pathogens, which the immune system can't see or get to, with resulting on-going inflammation.
Dehydration and inability of cells to flush wastes due to clogged elimination pathways, leading to cellular replication abnormalities.
Nutritional and absorption deficiencies.
Lack of exercise

Disrupted sleep, depression, anxiety, fear, and other negative emotions that cause the body to over-produce stress hormones and other compounds, in an effort to balance these conditions.

~~~~

"Be'champ found that the diseased acidic, low oxygen cellular environment is created by a toxic and nutrient deficient diet, toxic emotions, and a toxic lifestyle. He was able to scientifically prove that germs are the chemical by products and constituents of pleomorphic micro-organisms acting upon the unbalanced, malfunctioning, cell metabolism.

His findings demonstrate how cancer develops through the morbid changes of germs to bacteria, bacteria to viruses, viruses to fungal forms and fungal forms to cancer cells. He believed that the biological terrain of the being is the cause of the disease, not the germ itself. Germs are finding feeding material wherever our blood is acidic, fermenting, and where the supply of oxygen is blocked."
-Evita Ramparte, The Bliss of Cancer

Common Major Toxins

Microwave ovens- Radiation causes ionization, which is what occurs when a neutral atom gains or loses electrons. In simpler terms, "a microwave oven decays and changes the molecular structure of the food by the process of radiation." The radiation breaks down any vitamins and minerals in the food and changes their natural structure. The body cannot handle these irradiated molecules, and they eventually weaken the immune and digestive system, because of the harmful molecules and lack of proper nutrition. The research suggests that people who consume microwave-cooked food are more likely to develop stomach and intestinal cancers, have peripheral cellular tissue degeneration, and a gradual breakdown of the digestive and excretory system.

Acrylamide- Baked, fried or roasted starch food inevitably has acrylamide. Acrylamide is a chemical known to damage chromosomes, increase oxidative damage in tissues, injure nerve cells, and be a low grade carcinogen. Heavily cooking food, or microwaving, produces large amounts of acrylamides. French fries, potato chips and dark toast are some of the worst.

Heating the sugars in the starches oxidizes them to then react with the amino acid asparagine to form acrylamide. The higher the heat and longer the heating time the more acrylamide produced. Better options are to water sauté with a little oil or steaming.

Aspartame has been investigated as a possible cause of brain tumors, mental retardation, birth defects, epilepsy, Parkinson's disease, Fibromyalgia, and Diabetes, yet the FDA (that once sought to have aspartame removed from the market) has done nothing to regulate this toxic artificial sweetener.

Carrageenan- (found in most alternative milks) Even though it is a substance derived from red algae, that is also called carrageenan, several specific studies showed that food safe and approved carrageenan is contaminated with the non-approved degraded carrageenan. Furthermore, when you ingest the undegraded version, it actually starts to degrade in the gastrointestinal tract and in the liver and turn into a carcinogen, resulting in a serious inflammatory agent that also can cause intestinal abnormalities. Because of this reason and other studies conducted the World Health Organization's International Agency for Research on Cancer and the National Research Council of the United States both have determined that carrageenan is a carcinogen – a substance that causes cancer.

Heavy Metals- Our bodies are exposed to toxic metals from water supplies, cosmetics, medicine, commercial herbal supplements, hygiene products, dental fillings, vaccines, food and beverage storage, cookware, paints, cigarettes, and more. We're exposed to heavy metal toxins via ingestion, inhalation, and skin or eye contact. Once in the body, heavy metals multiply the production of harmful free radicals (by up to one million times) and cause deadly chain reactions. Heavy metals poison the body, impairing the function of cells, tissues, and organs, and can ultimately lead to cancer and countless other diseases.

Four metals that contribute to body toxicity are mercury, aluminum, lead, and cadmium. Lead is second, with mercury at a close third, and cadmium falls in as the eighth most toxic substance known to science. Aluminum, although not truly a heavy metal, is still an extremely poisonous substance that can accumulate in the body's tissues. Arsenic, the number one most toxic heavy metal, is very prevalent in some public water supplies.

Mercury- Both organic and inorganic mercury are highly toxic and can cause serious harm to the body. Inorganic mercury is used in thermometers, dental amalgam (fillings), batteries, barometers, skin-tightening creams, various pharmaceutical drugs (e.g. laxatives, diuretics, and antiseptics), and especially medicinal vaccines and pesticides. Inhalation of inorganic mercury vapors is the most common route of exposure, although ingestion, skin contact, and injection are possible routes.

Mercury is usually found in fish and other aquatic organisms but can also be detected in produce, livestock, processed grains, and dairy products. Most commonly, humans are exposed to mercury from vaccines (as elaborated upon in the Autism section), by eating contaminated fish or inhaling fumes from dental fillings. The use of mercury amalgam fillings for tooth cavities has generated much concern about this toxin. Once these fillings are in place, they continue to emit mercury vapors into the foods we eat, as we chew. Once swallowed, these mercury particles end up in the intestinal tract. The only "safe" amount of mercury in the body is none!

Sodium Fluoride and Pineal Gland Calcification- If seeking enlightenment through meditation, or perhaps looking to have a good night's rest, a healthy pineal gland is needed. Often referred to as the third eye, this small, pinecone-shaped endocrine organ, located in the brain, secretes and regulates melatonin, the hormone that regulates the circadian rhythms (our sleep-wake cycle) and certain sex hormones. The lack of it also contributes to thyroid problems that affect the entire endocrine system. The pineal gland is considered the physical link to the upper chakras or third eye for spiritual and intuitive openings.

As a calcifying tissue that is exposed to a high volume of blood flow, the pineal gland is a major target for fluoride accumulation in humans. This calcification process is caused by constant exposure to substances like fluoride which build up in the body over time. In fact, the calcified parts of the pineal gland (hydroxyapatite crystals) contain the highest fluoride concentrations in the human body, higher than either bone or teeth. Studies have found that calcified deposits in the pineal gland are associated with decreased numbers of functioning pinealocytes and reduced melatonin production as well as impairments in the sleep-wake cycle. This may also be a large contributor to severe migraine headache issues.

VOCs- Volatile Organic Compounds- Most of the toxins, we absorb from the air, are found indoors. Most paints (even latex paints) release chemicals known as Volatile Organic Compounds (VOCs) and these can be extremely toxic once airborne. VOCs have high vapor pressures and this allows them to evaporate quickly within the atmosphere. Millions of people are inhaling these toxic compounds on a daily basis. As VOCs build up in the body, they can lead to eye, nose, and throat irritation, headaches, loss of coordination, nausea, and damage to the liver, kidneys, and central nervous system. Some VOCs have even been shown to cause cancer in animals. VOC levels are generally estimated to be ten times greater in indoor environments than in outdoor spaces.

Mildew and mold reproduce via airborne spores that are constantly seeking more moisture. This is why mold is found in sections of a home that are likely to have damp surfaces such as walls (inside and out), cabinets, and any other poorly ventilated areas that can trap condensation and provide a breeding ground for mold.

Sick Building Syndrome occurs when inhabitants of a particular building report health symptoms seemingly linked to actual time spent in that building, however, no specific illness is pinpointed. Building Related Illness, on the other hand, characterizes an occupant's diagnosable condition that can be directly connected to the toxic agents pervading the air of the building. Building occupants complaining of temporary symptoms such as fatigue, dizziness, nausea, headache, dry cough, concentration difficulties, or eye, nose, and throat irritation are probably suffering from Sick Building Syndrome. In this situation, most symptoms subside after leaving the particular building.

Occupants suffering prolonged symptoms even after leaving a building are likely to have Building Related Illness. Symptoms of BRI include chest tightness, cough, chills, fever, and muscle aches. Poor indoor air quality is a major contributor of both conditions. Insufficient ventilation systems, toxic VOCs, and biological contaminants all contribute to a less than desirable environment.

Tap water/showers- Chlorinated tap water overwhelms the intestines with toxins and prevents essential nutrients from being absorbed into the body. Even if tap water is avoided, there are still toxins ingested simply by taking a shower. A hot shower can expose the body to toxic chemicals and showering for just fifteen minutes, can allow absorption of the same amount of toxins as drinking seven glasses of tap water. Moreover, the heat from a steaming shower causes skin pores to dilate and absorb even more of the toxins directly. Likewise, if lounging next to a pool on a hot day, the pores will dilate, and, when immersed in the pool, the skin can absorb high levels of chlorine through the wide-open pores.

Inhaling chlorine is a serious health risk since it can be absorbed directly into the bloodstream without being filtered by the kidneys. One study found that the consumption of chlorinated water significantly correlates to the onset of brain and colon cancer, and a higher risk for bladder and gastrointestinal cancer. A good shower filter and pure, filtered, drinking water from a high quality system, or spring water, or water bottled in glass are good choices!

Antibiotics are drugs that destroy bacteria or inhibit their growth and, while lifesaving in some situations, are possibly the most over-prescribed medication on earth. Antibiotics can kill beneficial bacteria, cause diarrhea and colitis, and lead to antibiotic resistance by bacteria, if overused. Very commonly, viral infections are misdiagnosed as bacterial infections. In these cases, patients receive a completely pointless dose of antibiotics. It's estimated that over fifty million pounds of antibiotics are prescribed every year. Whether the prescriptions are necessary or not, these antibiotic drugs are contaminating intestinal tracts and causing serious side effects.

This high incidence of food allergy or intolerance, which is greater than any other type of illness affecting mankind, has been associated with many disorders typically thought due to infection by bacteria. A classic example is ear infection in children. In one study 80% of children with ear infections have food reactivity. Casein in dairy products and gluten in wheat have been implicated in ear infections, tonsillitis, bronchitis and pneumonia, all routinely treated with antibiotics rather than simple dietary changes.

Prudent and judicious use of antibiotics can be lifesaving, while frequent overuse has contributed to thinning of the intestinal lining, overgrowth of yeast, susceptibility to invasion by parasites, poor absorption of nutrients, PMS, loss of sex drive, skin rashes, chronic constipation, recurring headaches, chemical and environmental sensitivities, poor memory/mental fuzziness, and subsequent immune and brain health issues and development of more food intolerances. Furthermore doctors in hospitals and clinics around the world are losing the battle against an onslaught of new, drug resistant, bacterial infections including staph, pneumonia, strep and other diseases that are costly and difficult if not impossible to treat.

"Good" bacteria (also referred to as friendly bacteria, microbiota, digestive flora, or intestinal flora) ideally, are passed on through mother's milk and take up residence in the colon shortly after birth. Trillions of these bacteria live, multiply, and help fight off infection. Although a small number of harmful bacteria may be present, they are far outnumbered by the good bacteria keeping them in check. However, increased antibiotics reduce the number of healthy bacteria, allowing bad bacteria/Candida to thrive.

If antibiotics kill off the friendly bacteria, Clostridium difficile are the most common, harmful bacteria to multiply in the colon. It produces a toxin that builds up in the colon, causes diarrhea, and severely damages the lining of the colon. Coconut water Kefir then becomes the best choice to counteract these bacteria. It's time to draw a distinction between antibiotics appropriate use and overuse!

EMFs- When electromagnetic radiation comes into contact with living matter, it causes ionization—the loss of electrons from atoms, which can cause chromosomal mutation or even cellular damage and death. If losing electrons negatively affects a cell, then it can also affect tissue, which will affect organs, and then entire bodily systems.

Losing electrons is much easier than gaining them. Watching TV, talking on cellular devices, working in an office with fluorescent lights—all these activities cause exposure to EMFs and can cause the body to lose electrons. Most

Americans saturate themselves by being surrounded with all the latest trendy, toys, technology, and other trivial "conveniences."

The body needs electrons to remain healthy and these daily, low doses of radiation, increases the risk of developing several cancers, including colon cancer. Radiation overstresses the colon and disrupts digestive processes, leading to abdominal pain, constipation, diarrhea, and cancer.

Many people are literally swimming in radiation every day. Urban areas in particular bombard the human body with toxic EMFs at home, work, school, and even outdoors. Toxic EMFs from cell phones and cellular towers and frequent/ prolonged use of cell phones can result in very serious health complications, such as brain tumors.

Parasites are organisms that live on or inside another organism called a "host," and can range from microscopic amoebas, bacteria, fungi, and viruses to large intestinal worms measuring several feet in length. These organisms operate on pure survival instinct, competing with the host for nutrients and excreting toxic waste that threatens health. In addition, parasites can cause further damage throughout the body as they migrate and encase themselves in hard protective shells, called bio-shields. Parasitic infestation can mimic the symptoms of an estimated fifty different diseases.

Biofilms are highly structured communities of microorganisms, often beneath layers of calcification that attach to one another and to surfaces. The microorganisms group together and form a slimy, polysaccharide cover. This layer is highly protective for the organisms within it, and when new bacteria are produced they stay within the slimy layer.

~~~~

"We have been so numbed down, living lives of quiet desperation and lining up like lambs to the slaughter, that few of us remember how to be fully alive, and feel constant, never ending energy and creative joy that borders on euphoria, how it is to know that you know and never doubt yourself." -Evita Ramparte

Colon Cleansing

The average person is walking around with anywhere from six to twelve pounds of undigested material fermenting in their intestines and colon. As these materials accumulate and subsequently begin to rot, the body wraps them in mucus to keep from being poisoned.

The impacted material is home base to four of the most dangerous threats to health. Number one, it is where toxins accumulate. Second, it is where virus and bacteria hide (when the immune system chases them out of the bloodstream) and where they breed and re-infect. Third, the impacted material is a fecal fortress for parasites to reside in. Fourth, it is an ideal garden for the overgrowth of undesirable flora such as Candida. By eliminating this impacted material, we are eradicating the home base to four of the largest assailants to health.

Two very important gut functions are assimilation and elimination. The colon is approximately three to five feet long. The walls are reasonably smooth and it is primarily an organ of elimination. If the colon is clogged with mucous and undigested material, the elimination process is impeded.
With health regimens involving the detoxification of the liver, kidneys, the bloodstream, and the lymph, if the colon is not cleaned first, these systems have nowhere to empty and back up. This creates a feeling of malaise known as a detox reaction, or healing crisis.

The intestines are approximately twenty feet long. Nature designed them with a maximum amount of surface area for absorption. The inside of the intestines is home to multitudes of villi, hundreds of finger-like projections, making the internal texture of the intestines much like a shag rug. When the villi become pasted down with mucus and impacted material they are less able to absorb nutrients from food or get maximum benefits from supplementation. Instead, toxins are being reabsorbed from the impacted material as it ferments.

By cleaning out the intestines (i.e. shampooing the shag rug), we are able get the maximum benefit out of the food we eat and the supplements we take. It is also a wonderful way to reduce bloat and relieve a chronically fatigued, tired feeling one gets from absorbing poisons into the bloodstream through the intestines, instead of nutrients. Vibrant health begins in the colon, and supplying the body with adequate fiber every day is highly beneficial to colon function and overall health. (See Daily Fiber Blend in Cleanse Ingredients section).

Integrative Medicine and Cleansing

Before disease is cured and health flourishes, nutritional deficiencies must be addressed, impurities cleansed from the 70 trillion cells in the body, opportunistic infections alleviated, immune health restored, and sound, new nutritional and lifestyle practices integrated. The sooner the better! As toxins are released and healthy new habits replace addictive food and lifestyle tendencies, suppressed emotions, and limiting negative mental attitudes arise to be acknowledged and worked with! Instead of numbing out or taking unneeded prescription drugs, real solutions are implemented by beginning to work with crafting our lifestyles, how we eat, move, think and supplement!

~~~~

"Following a correct diet and exercise plan as a remedy should not be labeled alternative or complementary medicine. It is simply the way all properly educated doctors should be practicing. Everything else should be called malpractice medicine. Offering patients drugs and surgical interventions without informing them that for most diseases, nutritional excellence and exercise are safer and more effective in the long run is not adequate informed consent to the use of medications. The risks of medicines are downplayed and they're supposed benefits greatly exaggerated by medical profession and drug industry who offer drugs as the panacea to all else." -Brian Clement

~~~~

Thank goodness for the wealth of information, excellent teachers, and amazing detoxification and longevity substances now available. Especially appreciated are the emerging new, and more aware, "Integrative" physicians, who focus on therapies that work with the whole being. By working with the underlying causes and wisely supporting the body's innate defenses, healing and detoxification mechanisms, real results are made and patients actually become healthier. By first determining the root cause of the illness, then working with the patient to combat the illness, while changing lifestyle factors, the maximum full recovery success rate is achieved.

~~~~

"Our society is experiencing a sharp increase in the number of people who suffer from complex, chronic diseases such as diabetes, heart disease, cancer, mental illness, and autoimmune disorders like rheumatoid arthritis. The system of medicine practiced by most physicians is oriented towards acute care, the diagnosis and treatment of trauma or illness that is of short duration and in need of urgent care, such as appendicitis or a broken leg. Unfortunately, the acute-care approach to medicine lacks the proper methodology and tools for preventing and treating complex, chronic disease.

Most physicians are not adequately trained to assess the underlying causes of complex, chronic disease and to apply strategies such as nutrition, diet, and exercise to both treat and prevent these illnesses in their patients. Functional medicine involves understanding the origins, prevention, and treatment of complex, chronic disease." -Mark Hyman (Institute of Functional Medicine)

~~~~

This "New Medicine" – sometimes called Functional, Complementary or Integrative Medicine, combines the best of modern science with natural healing traditions that have been proven effective over many generations. "Prescriptions" often include customized dietary and lifestyle changes, natural nutritional supplements and other complementary therapies that produce lifelong benefits. They focus on modalities that are safe, effective, often less expensive, and that do not harm.

These modalities can include:

Identify food allergies
Consuming mostly raw and organic with lots of alkalinizing green foods and juice
Nutritional supplementation: concentrated superfoods, essential fatty acids, amino acids, digestive enzymes/ other digestive supports, Vit. D, B12, antioxidants, cleansing and tonic herbs
Sleep, exercise, yoga
Meditation, positive thinking, self-awareness
Avoiding toxins including; tobacco, alcohol, soda, diet and energy drinks, preserved food, GMOs, sugar cookies, pies, cakes, candy, processed carbs, fast food, flour and chemicals!
Depending on health and symptomology different cleansing protocols/ formulations may be warranted.
Begin with detoxification of:
Bowel/colon, liver, kidneys, blood, heavy metals, Xenoestrogens, viruses.
Standard recommendation is to drink ½ body weight in lbs. of filtered or spring (non-plastic contained) water per day. (Full body weight in oz.'s, during cleanse).
Cleanses may include; coffee enemas, wheatgrass and vegetable juicing, infrared sauna, foot detox baths, lymphatic drainage, zeolites for heavy metals and Xenoestrogens, skin brushing, stress reduction, emotional and mental detox.
Treat all imbalanced systems: nutritional, hormonal, immune and mind/body.

Excellent detox centers are OHI- (Optimum Health Institute), Hippocrates Health Institute, Oasis of Hope-(Center for Integrative medicine) and more.

Be ready to experience the you, you have been looking for! As blockages leave on the physical/emotional plane space opens for a new life of Inspiration, Connection, Authenticity, Contribution and Fulfillment! Often, as we embark on the detoxification path, it becomes apparent we are also addressing blocks to our own consciousness/spirituality. When we truly commit to deep physical purification, refrain from addictive, numbing out habits and peel away toxic layers in the body, we open the door to clearing old, negative emotional patterns and mental programming.

Buddhists call these patterns afflictions and propensities, Hindus - Samscaras that can be repeated for lifetimes. To break free of the inertia of what no longer serves us and find ones true self, inner peace, authentic intimate relationships and real freedom requires emotional intelligence, letting go of addictions, and lifelong negative response patterns.

With practice, clear focus, commitment and the support of a healthy functioning body and clear mind, true fulfillment becomes life's journey. Now more than ever our own souls are calling for us to choose out of our personal limitations and the old paradigms addictions, barbaric factory farms, chemically laced, poisonous food supply, toxic media programming, stress caused hormonal disruptions, and drug/alcohol induced stupor…. to find the fulfillment that comes from realizing ones true self!

~~~~

"Without knowledge of the self, knowledge of outer things is like a string of zeros. Zeros are valueless until you place a numeral in front of them. In the same way, knowledge of the outer world may bring you great material benefit, but it cannot in itself bring satisfaction. As long as you are moving only on the outside, as long as you are looking for joy only in the outer world, you will never find it. But if you turn within you will experience the joy of the self, and then you will also find the same joy outside. Real happiness, real fulfillment, comes only when you discover the self." -Swami Muktananda, I Am That

~~~~

Often there is a grace, the feeling of being protected when we choose health on all levels. As we dedicate our lives to wholeness and service our intuition is activated to guide us on the way to true fulfillment! When we become present for our most important part in the Divine transformational plan our deepest joy, our most radiant being emerges to help us make a difference.

Happy, Healthy, Hormone Balance, Naturally

Hormone balance and health is a complex and multi-faceted endeavor that is still being discovered. Finding ways to keep hormones at healthy levels and in balance is of utmost importance because hormones are the master triggers of metabolism and tell cells what to do. Bio-identical hormone replacements and progesterone creams have been a miracle for many, yet if use stops, the body can revert back, so it is best to have healthy balanced hormones naturally! Hormones are the master switches of:
- Weight regulation and body fat composition
- Immunity function and anti-aging
- Energy levels and sex/health hormones

- Juvenile hormones (super health hormones)

Hormones important functions include protecting against cancer, improving memory, protecting the brain, promoting strong bones, speeding up healing time, increasing strength and focus, helping to adapt to stress, appetite stimulation, and mood improvement!

To accomplish its many tasks the endocrine system is composed of multiple glands and differing hormones. These include the:
Pineal, hypothalamus, pituitary, thyroid, parathyroid, thymus, adrenal, pancreas and ovaries/testes. Major hormones include: insulin, thyroid, growth, progesterone - the dominant female hormone, estrogens – (oppose testosterone and progesterone and regulate healthy metabolism) testosterone - dominant male hormone, DHEA, Vitamin D, adrenaline, norepinephrine, cortisol and leptin.

Imbalances can lead to: obesity, depression, cancer, diabetes, abnormal growth rate, aging, infertility, mood swings, heart disease, sleep apnea, high cholesterol, migraines, insomnia, acne...

Our current environment, life style and dietary factors can lead to shortages and imbalances. Some are:
Artificial light, medication - birth control pills, cholesterol medication, soy products, rancid oil, lack of healthy fats, pesticides, pollution (17,000 new chemicals were introduced into the environment since 1940), plastics, BPA, plasticizers (in drinking water bottles), lack of grounding/earthing (walking barefoot on the earth with the sky overhead...)

The liver can become compromised by fatty deposits of age-related estrogen, combined with phony estrogens - the Xenoestrogens from plastics, pesticides, herbicides etc. all sitting on the livers receptor sites. Xenoestrogens mimic healthy estrogen and clog up sites, preventing healthy metabolism.
Removing these deposits is fundamental to natural hormone balance and is done through the methylation process. These positively charged deposits are missing what's called a methyl group as they have un-bonded hydrogen in their composition. These can be attached to and dislodged with negatively charged methylators such as:
Betaine (in beets), DMG, MSM, Sam-e, Vitamins B6, B9, and B12
The bad estrogen is then removed with substances like citrus oil/peel, cruciferous vegetables with high Indole 3 carbonal like broccoli, defatted flax, calcium deglucarate, melatonin and beta-glucans.

~~~~

"I went to my doctor and he offered Prozac and birth control pills, but that just didn't feel right. I decided to apply my medical training to myself, and I discovered my cortisol level was insanely high (something my traditional doctors told me wasn't a big deal). Within one month, I had fixed the issue and felt enormously better. I took on my low thyroid next, and then my bad estrogens. I ate differently, exercised less, and took 3 supplements. I lost 25 pounds and graduated from couple's therapy. I was on to something! The solution to my problems became The Gottfried Protocol, and it has worked gloriously well on the 10,000+ people I've seen in the past 10 years." -Dr. Sarah Gottfried, The Hormone Cure

Three Treasures and Tonic Herbs

According to Taoist tradition, there are 3 fundamental energies housed in all living beings: Essence (Jing), Energy (Qi- Chi), and Spirit (Shen). The integration of these three energies constitutes our very existence, and they are considered treasures to be nourished protected and balanced. When these energies are sufficiently preserved and cultivated, health and longevity of the body, mind and spirit are achieved. Keeping them abundant should be the goal of every person, as to neglect the three energies is to neglect life itself.

Essence (Jing), the giver of Life, is the first Treasure. Jing is the concentrated, refined and regenerative energy we receive at our conception and is meant to last our entire lives. It is the foundation of our existence. Jing is the root energy of the body responsible for procreation, physical energy, sexual energy, creativity, longevity and youthfulness. Essence (Jing) is easily dissipated through excessive eating, drinking, sexual activity, work stress, lack of sleep and addictive behaviors. Becoming tired is natural, becoming exhausted is dangerous.
To preserve essence, Jing, the Taoists avoided extremes and sought to maintain balance in their lives and activities.

Energy (Qi or Chi), "the breath of life" is the second Treasure. While essence (Jing) is our deep reserve, Energy (Qi) is our day to day vitality. It is the energy we derive from the air we breathe and foods we eat. It is also our actual breathing. The deeper and more regulated our breathing, the healthier we become as blood and energy are more efficiently and deeply circulated to every cell of the body, leaving them more nourished and vitalized.

Spirit (Shen), "the light of life" is the third treasure. It is our mental, emotional and spiritual wellbeing as well as our connection to our higher self and the Divine. Spirit (Shen) is housed in the heart and provides us with feelings of peace, calm, and serenity. Shen gives us proper perspective on our life and our place in the universe. When the Spirit (Shen) is strong, attachment to the mundane dissipates and we become more childlike, awakened and at ease in the world around us. We become compassionate for and caring of others.

Over the past 5,000 years in China a unique and powerful system of cultivating health has developed with the use of herbs, numbering in the thousands. There are three distinguishable classes. Medicinal herbs are employed during sickness and are meant to be taken for short periods of time. General herbs are for harmonizing imbalances and can be part of an ongoing herbal program. Finally, there is a select group of about fifty herbs qualifying as tonic or "superior" herbs. This special class of herbs, when taken regularly, was considered by Taoists to be the substances from which health, longevity, and "immortality" could be achieved. In order for a herb to be considered a "Tonic" or "Superior" herb it must conform to the following:

1. Contain at least one of the Three Treasures
2. Provide a health benefit when consumed
3. Do no harm
4. No negative side effects when used properly
5. Can be taken for a lifetime

The organ system most closely related to the Taoist concept of Essence (Jing) is the Kidney/Adrenal complex. The Kidney essence energy has two components to it, Yin and Yang. Yin refers to the cooling replenishing aspect while Yang refers to the warming and kinetic aspect. As such, tonic herbs will either be classified as Yin tonics or Yang tonics.

The secret for maintaining optimal health is to have the proper balance between these two opposite and interdependent energies. Tonic herbs excel at this as Energy (Qi) is a Yang activity while blood is a Yin essence fluid.

Spirit-Shen Tonics are food for the soul and help to transcend the physical realm, allowing us to feel comfortable in one's own skin. According to Taoist philosophy they are associated with the heart energy and cultivate compassion, peace and love, helping us to evolve spiritually, to fulfill our highest callings. Some Spirit-Shen tonics are considered stabilizing agents, calming and grounding during times of stress. Radiant health is dependent upon one's ability to adapt appropriately and effectively to all the stresses one encounters in the course of one's life. Tonic herbs are said to provide "adaptive energy" which helps us handle stress much more easily.

The goal of tonic herbalism is to help the user of the tonic herbs to establish a harmony of body, mind and spirit which can result in a new level of wellbeing, a new level of health and happiness. This forms the foundation for a creative, successful life, as well as for true spiritual discovery, growth, and possibly, eventual mastery and enlightenment, so we may be the light in the world, fully living our highest purpose. Some favorite Tonic herbs are:

Astragalus is one of the most important herbs in the world and has been recognized as a superb and potent immune system tonic by modern researchers. Astragalus has been used for over 2000 years to strengthen the body as a whole and is believed by Oriental people to strengthen muscles and improve metabolic functions. Astragalus is said to have another effect on the "surface" of the body as it is used to tonify the "Protective Qi," known as Wei Qi in Chinese. This Protective Qi is a special kind of energy which circulates just under the skin and in the muscle. Recently there have been some Astragulus extract products scientifically proven to strengthen the Telomeres on the ends of DNA strands, directly influencing health, longevity, and youthfulness!

Dang Gui- (Tang Kuei Root) Also known as Angelica sinensis, it is used as a superb blood tonic. It is also an important blood-vitalizing herb (e.g. it improves blood circulation). Men use it as a muscle-building blood tonic, however, Dang Gui is most famous as a women's tonic, because women so often use it as a blood tonic and to regulate the female menstrual cycle.

Eucommia Bark is a superb Yang-Jing tonic, used to strengthen the back (especially the lower back), skeleton, and joints (especially the knees and ankles). Eucommia is believed to confer strength and flexibility to the ligaments and tendons. It is often used by martial artists, yoga practitioners, Qi Gung practitioners, and other athletes to strengthen the back, knees, and the entire body. It has been found to be very helpful at regulating blood pressure, especially high blood pressure.

Ginseng Root- Oriental Ginseng is one of the most famous and valued herbs used by mankind. Panax Ginseng is an energy tonic known to regulate the human energy system. It has been shown to be both stimulating and regulatory for both the central nervous system and to the endocrine system. It is the primary Qi tonic of Chinese tonic herbalism.

Ginseng helps a person to adapt to all kinds of stresses as well as enhancing endurance and resilience under stressful conditions. It has thus been termed an "adaptogenic" substance by scientific researchers. Ginseng is also used to tonify digestive and respiratory functions. Ginseng contains many active ingredients, but the most important are the saponins called ginsenosides. Ginsenosides specifically improve adaptability and are believed to help build muscle and endurance.

Goji berries/Lycium fruit are revered in Chinese Tonic herbalism as one of the top health sustainers, and as a promoter of cheerfulness and vitality. Regular consumption of this delicious fruit is traditionally believed to lead to a long and happy life, as it is known as a "secratagogue" or a substance with the ability to stimulate excretion of Human Growth Hormone from the pituitary gland. It is said prolonged consumption of Lycium will brighten the eyes and improve vision. Lycium fruit contains polysaccharides which have been demonstrated to strongly fortify the immune system, and it is also very rich in vitamin C and in B vitamins. Furthermore, it is the richest source of carotenoids, including beta carotene, of all known plants on earth, and is thus a powerful antioxidant!

Gynostemma Leaf is popularly believed in Asia to be an anti-aging, longevity herb. Gynostemma is generally reinforcing to overall health and has a strong anti-fatigue effect. It is also used throughout the Orient as a virtual "cure-all" and is a popular everyday tea. Gynostemma is a major adaptogenic herb, in the same league as Panax Ginseng, Siberian Ginseng, Reishi, Schizandra and Astragalus. In China, Gynostemma is widely believed to reduce oxygen deficiency at high altitudes, to improve digestion, to strengthen the mind, and to improve sexual functions. It also helps calm nerves and to ease pain.

The ultimate greatness of Gynostemma lies in its broad spectrum, adaptogenic quality, having double-direction activity in many areas. Constant consumption of Gynostemma tends to have a highly protective quality because it strengthens the adaptive capacity of the person, at every level of their life. The chemical parts responsible for the adaptogenic characteristic of Gynostemma are saponins called gypenosides.

He Shou Wu- (Fo Ti) Constant consumption of this famous "longevity herb," whose full name is Polygonum multiflorum, is said in the Orient to help return an aging person to youthfulness and to keep a young person young. It is an unsurpassed Yin-Jing tonic, as well as a major blood tonic. It is said to increase energy and to clean the blood. As an essence tonic, it is believed to be a powerful sexual tonic when consumed regularly. Polygonum is widely believed in China to increase sperm production in men and to increase fertility in women. It is used in almost all tonics believed in the Orient to nurture the hair and teeth. This herb has been consumed by almost every Taoist who has ever lived, and is fundamental to the practice of the Taoist inner arts.

Poria Mushroom is very widely used in Chinese herbalism. It is traditionally used as a Qi tonic to benefit the internal organs. It is a solid fungus found growing on the roots of old pine trees. It is mildly diuretic and sedative, and is considered to be highly nourishing. This herb has been widely used by Taoists through the centuries and was often consumed as a primary food source by

Taoist hermits. A special variety of Poria known as "Spirit Poria" is considered a premium Shen tonic herb. It is the part of the Poria mushroom containing the root of the old pine tree, upon which it has grown. Spirit Poria is said to benefit the heart, to nourish the Spirit and to lead to a long and happy life.

Rehmannia Root is said to be the "Kidney's own food." It is thus believed to be a Kidney tonic and longevity herb and is found in many common "antiaging" formulations for longevity and rejuvenation. It is also considered a premium blood tonic and is said to benefit sexual functions in men and women. The steamed variety is said to be warm in nature, and the steamed variety is the one considered tonic.

Rhodiola is thought to be helpful for reducing stress. This herb has been used for centuries throughout Asia and may also help to support a healthy immune system and alleviate symptoms of depression.

Schizandra Fruit is a famous tonic historically consumed by Chinese royalty and by Taoist masters. It is one of the few herbs containing all three treasures. Schizandra is renowned as a beauty tonic and is considered to be a youth preserving herb. It has been used for centuries to make the skin soft, moist and radiant. It is also said to be a powerful tonic to the brain and mind, and is believed in China to improve memory. It is also said to be an excellent sexual tonic giving increased sexual endurance and strength to the whole body when consumed regularly. It is used in many tonic formulations as an "astringent."

Schizandra, develops the primary energies of life, and generates vitality and radiant beauty when used regularly, over time. If used for 100 days successively, Schizandra is said to purify the blood, sharpen the mind, improve memory, rejuvenate the kidney energy (especially the sexual functions in both men and women), and cause the skin to become radiantly beautiful.

Siberian Ginseng is an incredibly important and popular tonic herb. Wild Eleutherococcus senticosis is found growing widely in Siberia, Mongolia and Northeastern China. It is famous as an adaptogenic herb, thus aiding in handling stress. It has been used for centuries to increase physical and mental endurance, to build blood and to improve memory. It is now widely used to regulate blood sugar levels, and is especially popular among athletes and those who work hard. It is perhaps the most popular herb in the world among martial arts practitioners.

Spring Dragon Tea- (Dragon Herbs) Gynostemma, Schizandra, Lycium-Goji, Austragalus, Eleuthero (Siberian Ginseng) Luo Han Guo.

Magical Medicinal Mushrooms

Wild Mushrooms grow from mycelial mats, which in nature, range throughout the ecosystem. Occasionally the mushroom pops up and releases spores which can fly away and make new colonies. It's hypothesized; mushrooms have a cognitive ability and can help improve our intelligence, as some of the mushrooms contain neuro-transmitters similar to what we have in our brain and digestive system.

Mushrooms and mushroom mycelium are also generously composed of serotonin's and other serotonin like compounds and the fine filament in the web like network of mycelium is obviously similar to the organization of human neurological pathways. As one side of the mushrooms neurological network repels a pathogenic invader it communicates to the rest of the network and likewise our immune systems can understand the immune response coded within the mycelium. Mycelium is the mushrooms actual mother and has anti-viral, anti-bacterial and immunomodulating properties.

Some mushrooms, such as Reishi, are excellent Candida yeast fighters. They readily consume yeast and have specific yeast defenses. Reishi are also reputed to confer spiritual awareness, being of great benefit to the pituitary gland. Another mushroom known as Lions Mane has been found to have compounds able to regrow nerves and the myelin sheath covering. Some popular ones are:

Cordyceps sinensis- Himalayan mountain peoples have traditionally used Cordyceps to enhance their performance during strenuous, high altitude activities. Recently, physical fitness enthusiasts and professional athletes have discovered that Cordyceps provides the cardio-enhancing effect of increasing oxygen uptake, thereby supporting higher endurance levels. Cordyceps is one of the absolute superstars of the Chinese tonic herbal system. It is an extremely effective and powerful life-enhancing agent, ranking right up there with Ginseng and Reishi. It is said to build sexual and physical power, mental energy, the immune system and is universally believed in the Orient to prolong life.

Lion's Mane- *(Hericium erinaceus)* This beautiful species, appearing as a white waterfall of cascading icicles, is found on broad leaf trees and logs. The subject of recent studies on nerve regeneration it has been proven this tasty mushroom can regenerate brain cells in individuals who have lost cells due to stress and other causes. Lion's Main mushroom has been used traditionally by Buddhist monks in China to enhance brain power.

Reishi- *(Ganoderma lucidum* s.l.) grows throughout the world, and is found primarily on hardwood trees. This species, used for more than two millennia in Asia, is the most revered herbal substance in Asia, ranking as the elite provider of the realization of radiant health, longevity and spiritual attainment. It ranks in Asia with Ginseng, Rhodiola, and Cordyceps as a pre-eminent tool in the quest for radiant health. It has maintained this position for at least 3000 years, and its reputation is only increasing.

Numerous legends provide a rich and extensive record of Reishi in Asian society. It has long been a favorite tonic food supplement by the Chinese Royal family and virtually anyone who could obtain it. Reishi was particularly revered by the followers of the Taoist tradition as the "Elixir of Immortality." Taoists have continuously claimed Reishi promotes calmness, centeredness, balance, inner awareness and inner strength. They have used it to improve meditative practices and to protect the body, mind and spirit, so the adept could attain both a long and healthy life and "spiritual immortality" (enlightenment).

Chaga- *(Inonotus obliquus)* has been embraced by Eurasians for centuries. Found throughout boreal forests, it grows primarily on birch trees. Studied and treasured worldwide for its health-enhancing, anti-inflammatory and anti-oxidant properties, Chaga is a unique species, and the focus of recent and ongoing scientific research. It has a mild, pleasing flavor and excellent health benefits!
Shitake mushroom is a potent immune modulating herb. It contains the beta-glucan type of polysaccharides have been found to bolster the immune response of humans. Shitake helps reduce blood lipids and "bad" cholesterol. Shitake is widely used as a food, and is available as a food supplement.

Agaricus Mushroom is not a traditional Asian herb. It is a Brazilian rainforest herb which has won huge acceptance in Asia and is now commonly incorporated into Chinese tonic herbal formulations, in China and Japan. Of all known, natural immune substances, it is among the premier immune system tonics. It is the richest source in the world of a type of polysaccharide known as *beta-glucans*, which has been solidly established to be among nature's most potent immune potentiating substances. Agaricus has *double-direction activity* on the immune system. In other words, it may be used to bolster a deficient immune system, as occurs in cases involving infections, or Agaricus may be used to moderate an excessive system, as occurs in cases of autoimmune disease and allergies. In Japan, Agaricus is considered a "cure-all" herb.

Maitake Mushroom has gained a place in tonic herbalism due to its broad spectrum tonic benefits, similar to Agaricus and Reishi. Like Agaricus, it is primarily beneficial to the immune system, having double-direction activity on the entire immune system. It has been the subject of studies worldwide and is known for supporting normal cell growth. Rich in 1,3 - 1,4 and 1,6 beta-D glucans, Maitake is a delicious, edible species, with a long history of traditional use.

Ayurveda- the Ancient "Science of Life" from India

Ayurveda is the premier holistic healing system from India. Translated from Sanskrit as "the science of life" or "the knowledge of longevity" it is a volumous collection of interrelated practices that oversee literally every aspect of a person's health and lifestyle. Ayurveda is likely the oldest continuing healing system on the planet, with evidence of written records going back 5,000 years and an oral tradition going back thousands of years previous.

In Ayurveda, mind, body and spirit are inextricably entwined. Ayurveda and Yoga are sister practices, two sides of the same coin. Ayurveda is the physical/health/medical side of the philosophies while yoga is the science of spiritual development. Ayurveda is a complete approach to health and lifestyle management, a system incorporating diet, exercise, life activity routines, psychotherapeutic practices, massage and botanical medicine, which is the foundation of Ayurvedic therapeutics. Ayurveda works with the 5 elements; ether, air, fire, water and earth, which are condensed into 3 body types or "doshas," Pitta, Vata and Kapha. Ayurveda works with a vast body of knowledge to define, understand and maintain equilibrium of these elements.

One of the many great books on Ayurveda is, The Way of Ayurvedic Herbs- by Khalsa and Tierra. Some favorites, of the many wonderful herbs from Ayurveda, are listed next. For great sources for Ayurvedic herbs and formulations please check the Resources section of the Longevity Source website!

Amalaki- Amla is a small, very sour fruit that is the most widely used general rejuvinative in Ayurvedic formulas. The fruit is a spectacular source of vitamin C content, 20 to 30 times more than of oranges, making it also a powerful anti-oxidant. It is a superb tonic for the eyes, especially with nearsightedness and cataract treatment, as well as a tonic for the blood, bones, liver and heart. It enhances production of red blood cells strengthening teeth, hair and nails while regulating blood sugar. Amla is also a "frontline" anti-inflammatory herb, being used for a wide variety of inflammatory conditions.

Arjuna (Terminalia arjuna) is the foremost rejuvenative for the heart. It strengthens and tones the circulatory system and promotes proper function of the heart muscles. Arjuna's strengthening and toning actions help maintain healthy blood pressure already within the normal range. It is also used to help maintain healthy cholesterol levels and to support healthy coagulation. Arjuna is traditionally used to promote emotional balance for those experiencing grief and sadness. It is said to mend a 'broken heart' and to impart courage and strengthen the will. (medium taste)

Ashwagandha (Withania somnifera) is one of the most highly regarded and commonly used adaptogens in the Ayurvedic pharmacopoeia. Maximizing the body's ability to resist stress, it enables the body to reserve and sustain vital energy throughout the day while promoting sound, restful sleep at night. It is considered one of the best herbs for calming Vata and for revitalizing the male reproductive system.

Used by both men and women, it maintains proper nourishment of the tissues, particularly muscle and bone, while supporting proper function of the adrenals. This potent herb is used to promote muscle strength and to support comfortable joint movement. It is also used to maintain potency and a healthy libido, for it is said to bestow upon its user the vitality and strength of a horse. (good, semi-sweet flavor)

Brahmi/Bacopa (Bacopa monniera) is an excellent rejuvenative for the mind and nervous system. It is one of two herbs commonly known as the legendary "Brahmi" of the ancient Ayurvedic texts (the other being Brahmi/Gotu Kola). This amazing herb has been used for centuries to promote memory, intelligence and concentration. Bacopa supports the proper function of the brain and nerves, bringing balance to the nervous system while promoting clarity and awareness. It is also commonly used externally in a base of sesame oil as nurturing massage oil that calms and soothes the mind and nerves. (medium taste)

Haritaki (Terminalia chebula) is one of the three ingredients in the Ayurvedic super formula Triphala, and is considered to be one of the best herbs for balancing Vata dosha. Supporting the body's natural cleansing process, it gently removes accumulated natural toxins in the gastrointestinal tract. As a rejuvenative, it strengthens and nourishes the tissues and supports the proper function of the colon, lungs, liver and spleen. Haritaki is traditionally used as a remedy for all Vata-related imbalances. It maintains regular elimination, helps promote healthy body mass, and supports comfortable and complete digestion. In India, Haritaki is highly revered, as it is believed to increase energy, intelligence and awareness. (fairly bitter taste)

Guduchi (Tinospora cordifolia) The health promoting powers of this herb were so respected by the authors of the ancient Ayurvedic texts that they called it 'Amrita' or 'Divine Nectar'. A powerful nutritive tonic, Guduchi is one of the best herbs for balancing Vata and pitta. It has the unusual characteristic of being heating while simultaneously removing excess pitta from the body. This heat burns accumulated natural toxins, purifying the liver, kidneys, joints and blood. It also helps soothe the skin and promotes a clear, healthy complexion. Guduchi strengthens the tissues, bolsters immunity and promotes vitality while calming the mind and supporting proper function of the nervous system. It is also traditionally used to promote longevity and to support healthy reproduction.

Gokshura (Tribulus terrestris) is a rejuvenating tonic for the genitourinary system. A cooling and nourishing herb, gokshura soothes the membranes of the urinary tract while promoting the healthy flow of urine. It supports proper function of the kidneys, bladder and prostate. It tones the male reproductive system promoting virility, control and the healthy production of sperm. In women, Gokshura rejuvenates the uterus and helps promote fertility. It calms the nerves, strengthens the body and is balancing for all doshas. (bitter taste)

Holy Basil (Tulsi) has been revered as the most sacred herb in India for over five thousand years. Holy Basil is traditionally used as an Ayurvedic adaptogenic supertonic to support the brain, nervous, and respiratory systems. Holy Basil contains antioxidant compounds and restorative phyto-chemicals and is known to be safe to take on a daily basis.

Holy Basil supports the immune system and a healthy inflammatory response in the lungs and respiratory tract. It produces natural expectorant-like qualities and may be used to help support healthful lungs and sinuses, immune-response, and normalized esophageal passageways. Holy Basil is thought to support healthful blood viscosity. In addition, it may support healthful cholesterol and triglyceride levels already in normal range, and is an overall cardio-supportive herb.

One of the most well researched effects of the Holy Basil plant is its effects on stress. It acts as an adaptogen, increasing the body's ability to adapt to difficult circumstances. It helps support healthful adrenal response and cortisol levels, and aids in supporting neurotransmitter activity in the brain. It may also help improve stamina, memory, and emotional balance. As such, it has been used to support a positive mental outlook, optimal energy and response to stress.

Mucuna Puriens, also known as Kapikacchu seed powder or Tribulus is a nutritive tonic, commonly used in Ayurveda as an aphrodisiac and to support proper function of the reproductive system. It increases sexual energy and strengthens and tones the reproductive organs. In men, Mucuna supports potency, stamina and control. In women it promotes a healthy libido and fertility. The vitality bestowed by this herb nourishes the entire body and calms the nerves making it an excellent rejuvenative for Vata. It is also a natural source of levadopa (L-dopa) which is an essential precursor to the neurotransmitter dopamine, often absent in Parkinson disease cases. (very bitter taste)

Shatavari (Asparagus racemosus) is a rejuvenating herb that cools the body and strengthens and nourishes the tissues. As a nutritive tonic it encourages the healthy production of milk in lactating mothers and the healthy production of semen in would be fathers. It is also useful during menopause and for women who have had hysterectomies. Shatavari supports a healthy immune system and assists in both physical and mental digestion. Its unctuous quality soothes and nurtures membranes of the lungs, stomach, kidneys and reproductive organs. Sattvic (pure, harmonious) in nature, Shatavari calms the mind and promotes love and devotion. (mellow flavor)

Vidari Kanda (Ipomoea digitata) is a nutritive tonic that is rejuvenating for both body and mind. As is the case with many nourishing herbs, it has a special affinity for supporting the reproductive system. In men it supports healthy production of semen. In women it supports healthy menstruation and healthy lactation. In both sexes it is a strengthening aphrodisiac that supports fertility and vitality. Vidari Kanda is also traditionally used to pacify excess Vata.

Beneficial Nutrients

Chlorella is green algae. The name Chlorella derives from two Latin words meaning leaf (green) and small, referring to the unusually high content of chlorophyll (the highest of any known plant). This fresh-water, single celled microscopic plant contains a host of health building nutrients including vitamins, minerals, dietary fiber, nucleic acids, amino acids, enzymes, and more.
It has been called the "great normalizer," balancing out of balance body functions back in. Chlorella promotes growth in young people, which is believed to be related to Chlorella's capacity to stimulate the healing process in the body and stifle many diseases. This is most likely related to its nucleic acid content which accelerates growth in young people and promotes repair of damaged tissue in mature animals and humans.

Chlorella has a beneficial effect on body cells by strengthening metabolic pathways and Chlorella has an abundance of RNA and DNA which are associated with anti-aging. Chlorella promotes healthy cell reproduction, reduces cholesterol and increases hemoglobin levels. Because of its broad nutritional and detoxifying profile, Chlorella promotes the repair of bodily organs and tissues that have been injured or otherwise damaged.

Numerous research projects in the USA and Europe indicate Chlorella can also aid the body in the breakdown of persistent hydrocarbon and metallic toxins such as DDT, PCB, mercury, cadmium and lead, while strengthening the immune system response. The fibrous materials in Chlorella also improve digestion and promote the growth of beneficial aerobic bacteria in the stomach.

Organic Wheatgrass/Kamutgrass- Clinics all over the world have been set up to administer the miraculous juices extracted from sprouted wheat plants. People report that the intensive cleansing, which its chlorophyll and enzymes provide, is unsurpassed in its abilities to stimulate the immune response and initiate healing.

Organic Spirulina- An amazingly complete source of highly digestible, vegetarian protein, rich in B vitamins, particularly B-1, B-2, B-3, B-6, and more importantly, the richest source of B-12 in nature. Spirulina has shown promise in the treatment of impaired immunity, protein deficiencies and eating disorders.

Omega Zen oil + EPA is derived from natural marine plant sources. It is completely vegan and free of contaminants, with no marine odor or after taste. It is micro-cultured and thus grown under controlled conditions, so as to insure a very clean product. It is a highly concentrated, extra strong omega-3 DHA + EPA with twice the active ingredients of these two critical omega-3 fatty acids. It is a leading nutraceutical for enhanced cognitive and cardiovascular function.

O-Mega-Zen3 + EPA is produced in a soft vegan capsule, made from seaweed, which contains non-GMO starch, glycerin, purified water, maltitol (0.028 mgs per capsule). It contains no gluten, artificial colors or flavors, preservatives, dairy, yeast or wheat and does not contain any animal material.
Contains DHA (Docosahesaenoic Acid) 200+mg and EPA (Eicosapentaenoic Acid as Marine Microalgae Oil) 100+mg.

Aged Garlic extract contains stable, water-soluble sulfur substances, including S-allyl mercaptocysteine (SAMC) and S-allyl cysteine (SAC), which have high bioavailability with about 98 percent absorption into the blood. Also present are some oil-soluble sulfur compounds, flavonoids, a phenol known as allixin and other nutrients, including selenium. The aging process eliminates odor-causing components, resulting in the truly odorless Kyolic® Aged Garlic Extract containing safe, stable, bioavailable and beneficial compounds including ones known to destroy pathogenic organisms.

Rooibos tea from the Cape of South Africa is famous for its stunning red color and concentration of antioxidants and polyphenols. It is a great tasting, naturally caffeine-free tea, which is low in tannins (a substance known to affect the metabolism by decreasing absorption of certain nutrients like iron and protein) so it may be safely consumed all day. Rooibos is fermented to liberate its broad spectrum of phytonutrients, including Aspalathin, Quercetin, Orientin and Chrysoerio, is rich in minerals, and boosts glutathione levels. Scientific studies also show Rooibos Tea is naturally high in Super Oxide Dismutase (SOD), an outstanding antioxidant.

Pau De Arco is the bark from a tree called Taheebo, which grows mostly in Brazil and Argentina. Indigenous people noticed the Pau De' Arco tree did not rot, even when dead. It contains intrinsic chemical factors which fight fungus and mold, even in some of the wettest environments on earth. This is likely how and why indigenous people started using the bark medicinally. It makes an excellent and power-packed immune boosting tea, especially when combined with Una De Gato, the combo being traditionally called Shapibo tea.

Una De Gato or Cat's Claw- Uncaria tomentosa grows as a vine in the Amazon, where the root bark is stripped off and made into herbal teas. Cat's Claw is probably the most revered medicinal herb in all of South American herbalism due in large part to its alkaloids. Cat's Claw is regularly used in South America instead of pharmaceutical and over-the-counter drugs, in addition to being one of the most delicious and medicinally effective teas.

Horsetail (Equisetum arvense) is a primitive, perennial plant, closely related to the fern. It has hollow stems, tooth-like leaves and shoots sometimes compared to asparagus. When the plant dries, the branches feather outward and health promoting silica crystals form inside the stems.

Nettle- Urtica dioica is a flowering plant with leaves and stems covered in bristly hairs, causing a painful "stinging" sensation when touched. Throughout history stinging nettle has been used for various purposes. Native Americans used the plant's fibers to make rope, and boiled the roots and leaves for food. It was also used as a folk remedy for joint health and seasonal challenges. It contains vitamins A and C, and minerals potassium, calcium and manganese along with antioxidant flavonols, phytosterols, lignans and more.

Mamaki- (Hawaiian Nettles) is Hawaii's most delicious and nutritious native, tonic herb. This ancient native Hawaiian plant evolved in the islands prior to the Polynesians arrival in Hawaii, only grows in Hawaii and is found nowhere else in the world. The premium leaves are hand plucked from the tips of the plant and make a natural healing herbal tea and tonic. The Mamaki botanical also produces edible white berries, annually, that grow along its branches.

Mamaki is best known as a refreshing herbal tea, and is reputed to contain healing properties as a tonic for its numerous health and medicinal benefits. It is known as a herbal remedy for general debilities, lowering high blood pressure, reducing cholesterol, and cleansing toxins from the blood, as well as relieving stress and fatigue. It was, and is to this day, used for stomach problems, colon problems, liver troubles, bladder problems and irregular bowels. It has also been credited with helping maintain balance for diabetes, with some people.Hawaiian Mamaki is naturally cholesterol and caffeine free. People consume the leaves raw or cooked, as it is a nutritious green leafy vegetable. The berry and the tea have mild laxative properties as well as being useful to treat yeast infections for women.

Olena'- Cucuma longa (yellow variety) and Cucuma aromatica (orange, milder variety) are best known throughout the world as Turmeric, and are one of the two dozen or so, food and medicinal plants brought to Hawai`i by early Polynesian settlers in their voyaging canoes.  In Hawai`i, `Olena means yellow and it is `Olena's bright yellow rhizome which is precious. In tropical India, turmeric is widely cultivated as a dye, as a spice and potent Ayurvedic healing herb. Its use enhances the immune system by purifying the blood and being anti-bacterial. Olena also lessens morning stiffness and joint swelling, is known as a great antioxidant and is anti-inflammatory.

Stevia pure plant leaf all natural extract is super sweet, with no calories, carbs or sugars. Due to stevia's lack of a fully rounded flavor it excels as a flavor extender to stretch small amounts of other sweeteners, or in combination with citrus.

Superfood Heaven Glossary

Maca is enzyme-rich, with a pleasant malty taste, suitable for smoothies, raw desserts and juices, or in water/chai tea. Maca is known as Brazilian Ginseng, has a reputation as a powerful strength and stamina enhancer, as well as a libido-enhancing food-herb stretching back into prehistory. Like goji berries and ginseng, maca is a powerful adaptogen, which means it has the ability to balance and stabilize the body's systems (cardiovascular system, nervous system, endocrine system, musculature, lymphatic system, etc.).

As an adaptogen, maca can provide more energy if it is needed, but will not over stimulate the body. Adaptogens also boost immunity and increase the body's overall vitality by 10-15% according to most studies. Rather than addressing a specific symptom, adaptogens are used to improve the overall adaptability of the whole body to diverse and challenging situations and stress.

.

Cacao- David Wolfe is the leading authority on raw cacao, (Naked Chocolate is a great book by him) and he is the original introducer to the US of this incredible superfood. The raw cacao bean is one of nature's most fantastic superfoods, due to its mineral content and wide array of unique and varied properties. Raw cacao (unprocessed chocolate) is the number one source of magnesium of any food on the planet and contains one of the highest concentrations of antioxidants of any food in the world. Cacao is exceptionally rich in: chromium, anandamide (the bliss chemical) theobromine, manganese, zinc, copper, Omega-6 fatty acids, PEA, tryptophan, serotonin, etc. Cacao is also a super-natural energy enhancer!

Hemp Seeds are the most nutritious seed in the world and one of the most potent foods available, supporting optimal health and wellbeing. Hemp seeds are a complete protein and have a concentrated balance of proteins, essential fats, vitamins and enzymes, combined with a relative absence of sugar, starches and saturated fats. Raw hemp provides a broad spectrum of health benefits, all 20 amino acids, including the 9 essential amino acids.

Hemp seeds have a high protein percentage of the easily digestible, simple proteins, to strengthen immunity and fend off toxins as well as being nature's highest botanical source of essential fatty acid, with more essential fatty acid than flax, or any other nut or seed oil. It has a perfect 3:1 ratio of Omega-6 Linoleic Acid and Omega-3 Linolenic Acid – for cardiovascular health and general strengthening of the immune system. Hemp also contains a rich source of phytonutrients, the disease-protective element of plants with benefits to protect immunity, the bloodstream, tissues, cells, skin, organs and mitochondria.

Chia Seeds have been used for centuries, for a host of different reasons. When these seeds are hydrated in water, the seeds shell opens and absorbs up to nine times its volume in water. This then forms a gel, which is called chia seed gel. The gel helps keep the body hydrated and is also 90% soluble fiber, which is highly beneficial for the digestive track.

The seeds have twice the protein of any other seed or grain and five times the calcium of milk. It also has boron, which is trace mineral that helps transfer calcium into bones and Omega 3 and Omega 6, which are essential oils for the body. These seeds are also known to be an effective way to control the appetite.

Black Sesame seeds have very high amounts of calcium, magnesium and copper. Copper is well known for helping relieve some of the pain and swelling of Rheumatoid Arthritis and is effective in many anti-inflammatory systems. Black sesame has been used for thousands of years in Chinese medicine as a Kidney tonic, which is related to youth, vigor and sexuality. Black sesame is also used to promote regularity and, due to its high phytosterol content, reduce blood levels of cholesterol, enhance immune response, help with Asthma and other respiratory challenges.

Carob- Raw carob powder has way more nutrition and flavor than the usual roasted variety. Besides adding a wonderful, complimentary, flavor to cacao, with a nutritionally complimentary balancing effect, raw carob has more calcium and potassium, to balance perfectly with cacao's high levels of magnesium and sulfur. Also carobs sweet flavor helps decrease the bitterness of cacao. One part carob to 2 parts cacao is an ideal blend ratio.

Coconut Water Cultured Kefir can be made from raw or packaged varieties of coconut water. Kefir has many benefits including better digestion of fats, proteins and carbohydrates, and has been known for thousands of years for its anti-aging and immune enhancing properties. A good idea after antibiotic use!

Kefir is an ancient cultured food rich in amino acids, enzymes, calcium, magnesium, phosphorus and B vitamins. Coconut water kefir is full of beneficial microbes and powerful metabolites found in coconut water. It can provide a multitude of benefits, like:

Control opportunistic yeast growth, like Candida.

Guard against food-borne pathogens with seven different strains of probiotic bacteria and yeast.

Lactobacillus Kefir alone was found to fight the toxins produced by Clostridium difficile, a bacterium that contributes to chronic and sometimes deadly diarrhea. Because C. difficile is increasingly resistant to antibiotics, C. difficile infection is life threatening. Kefir may fight cancer and boost immunity, with probiotic chemical messages. All this and so much more!

Unlike yogurt, kefir can actually colonize the intestinal tract and is simple and fun to make at home. Using raw, fresh coconut water or packaged water, super healthy Kefir is easy to make, with many different flavor options such as Acai berry, ginger-cinnamon etc. Different probiotic foods like raisins or figs are wonderful inputs! Kefir Starter contains multiple beneficial bacteria. Each packet (from Body Ecology) makes an average of seven generations, with 3 to 4 oz. of previous batch, used to make one new quart of delicious Kefir liquid.

Sauerkraut- Healthy human colons contain many beneficial bacteria, which feed on the waste left over from digestion. Without these beneficial bacteria the human digestive system becomes home to harmful parasites and yeasts, resulting in Candida conditions.

Sauerkraut provides a high density source of a wide range of beneficial, live bacteria which assist in the digestive process. Consuming a serving of sauerkraut can give the body more of a health boost than many of the expensive probiotic drinks and supplements sold in stores.

To gain the most benefits from sauerkraut, its best to purchase unpasteurized or freshly made, or learn how to make your own. If you want to explore more recipes for making sauerkraut and other fermented dishes, an excellent place to start is with Sandor Ellis Katz's, Wild Fermentation: The Flavor, Nutrition and Craft of Live Culture Foods. Also Summer Bock on Fermented Foods in Resources section. See Raw Coconut Kefir and Sauerkraut in the recipe section of Longevity Source.

Himalayan Pink Crystal salt is 250 million year old salt, hand-mined with respect for nature, the environment, the workers, and the salts inherent bio-energetic qualities. Table salt or sodium chloride is extremely toxic. Some table salt contains aluminum hydroxide (a toxic metal and a known cause of Alzheimer's). Regular table salt is usually iodized. Naturally occurring iodine is essential, but added iodine is considered a toxic metal. The problem with sea salt is many of the oceans waters are polluted with heavy metals like lead, cadmium, arsenic, mercury and more. Oil disasters and leaking tankers pollute our oceans even more making sea salt less beneficial than it was in the past.

Himalayan Salt contains electrolytes in its 84 minerals and trace elements. Electrolytes such as sodium, calcium and potassium help restore the bodies' fluids. Electrolytes are what cells (especially nerve, heart and muscles) use to maintain voltages across cell membranes and to carry nerve impulses and muscle contractions across themselves and to other cells. Electrolytes have to be continually replaced whenever we sweat.

Super Berries

Açaí- (Euterpe Precatoria - pronounced ah-sigh-ee) is a unique, dark, purple berry which grows high up in the Acai palm trees native to Central and South America, and is found predominantly in the Amazonian Rain Forest. Acai berries contain Vitamin C, and are an excellent source of polyphenols, including rutin, anthocyanins, and catechins. Acai is naturally rich in ellagic acid and has up to 33 times the antioxidant content as red wine grapes. It has superior antioxidant protection and cardiovascular support, while supporting a healthy immune and inflammatory response. Acai has a mild blackberry flavor and is available frozen, unsweetened, or as freeze dried powder. Excellent in smoothies/desserts with dates and/or coconut sugar. More outstanding super berries are:

Camucamu Berry is grown in the Amazon and contains 30-60 times the vitamin C content of oranges and is up to 20% vitamin C by weight. Camu berries also have a full complement of minerals and amino acids that can aid in the absorption of vitamin C. Because of its food form, with bio-flavonoids and other phytochemicals, Camu berries are far more effective than synthetic vitamin C.

Mulberries when dried are extra delicious, sweet, and a rare food source of concentrated Resveratrol along with vitamin C fiber and protein.

Maqui Berry- With a mellow berry flavor and deep purple color, they are the highest known antioxidant berry, with double the ORAC value of Acai. Known to help with DNA strength, anti-aging and brain function, Maqui berries are the staple food to the Mapuche Indian tribe of Chile, one of the healthiest and longest living peoples in the world.

Goldenberry is best known as Poha berry which is easily cultivated in many of Hawaii's gardens. With a refreshing, sweet-sour flavor, it is a good source of vitamin A and C and bioflavonoids. Best fresh or sun dried. Other excellent berries include Aronia, Amla…

~~~~

"Health care costs are reaching a tipping point. They are not financially sustainable for the government or for many families. Most large businesses are self-insured, and this is coming right off their bottom line. I say, "If 75% of the $2.8 trillion in health care costs are for chronic diseases, which can often be prevented and even reversed by making comprehensive lifestyle changes, this can be a third alternative. By teaching people how to change their lifestyles, we can make better care available to more people at significantly lower costs—and the only side-effects are good ones." -Dean Ornish MD

Super Healthy Foods

"Folly in the getting of our food is nothing new. And yet the new follies we are perpetrating on our industrial food chain today are of a different order. By replacing solar energy with fossil fuel, by raising millions of food animals in close confinement, by feeding those animals foods they never evolved to eat (GMO corn laced with glyphosate and antibiotics) and by feeding ourselves foods far more novel than we even realize, we are taking risks with our health and the health of the natural world that are unprecedented."
-Michael Polan, Omnivores Dilemma

~~~~

Aloe Vera Juice- The aloe vera plant contains over 200 biologically active components. Aloe Vera is one of the best sources of germanium; a trace element which stimulates cellular purification and regenerates cell functions. Germanium is water soluble, is easily absorbed by the body and the excess is expelled through the urine, carrying heavy metals out of the body. Aloe Vera is also an excellent cleanser which helps with blood purification.

Its high choline content helps treat liver diseases and it prevents fat accumulation in the liver, thus avoiding fatty liver problems. Choline is useful in the prevention of liver diseases such as cirrhosis, cancer, and liver degradation, caused by toxins. Aloe is excellent in supporting a healthy digestive system and regularity, helps promote normal muscle and joint function and provides increased immune and antioxidant support.

Raw Coconut Oil preserves the live enzymes, lauric acid, and all the other immune system building nutrients, which richly abound in this oil. It has been described as the "healthiest oil on Earth" and is composed mainly of medium-chain-fatty-acids (MCFA) with 86.5% saturated fatty acids, 5.8% monounsaturated fatty acids, and 1.8% polyunsaturated fatty acids. It is the world's only low-calorie fat! Of the saturated fatty acids, coconut oil is primarily 44.6% lauric acid, 16.8% myristic acid, and 8.2% palmitic acid.

In comparison to most oils, coconut oil has a long shelf life, of up to three years, which is due to its being the most stable of all oils, slow to oxidize, and thus resistant to rancidity. Coconut oil is one of the best sources of natural nutrition for hair as it helps to make a healthy growth of hair and provide a shiny complexion. It is an excellent conditioner and helps in the re-growth of damaged hair, providing the essential proteins required for nourishing damaged hair.

Coconut oil is excellent massage oil for the skin as well. It acts as an effective moisturizer on all types of skin including dry skin. The benefit of coconut oil on the skin is comparable to mineral oil. Coconut oil is a safe solution for preventing dryness and flaking of skin, as well as sagging of skin, which normally becomes prominent with age. Coconut oil also helps in treating various skin problems including psoriasis, eczema and other skin infections. It also helps in preventing premature aging and degenerative diseases due to its antioxidant properties.

There is a misconception spread among many people coconut oil is not good for the heart. This is because it contains a large quantity of saturated fats. However, coconut oil is beneficial for the heart as it contains about 50% lauric acid, which helps in preventing various heart problems, including high cholesterol levels and high blood pressure.

Coconut oil is very useful in reducing weight. It contains short and medium-chain fatty acids to help in taking off excessive weight. It is also easy to digest and helps with the functioning of the thyroid and enzymes systems. The saturated fats present in coconut oil have anti-microbial properties and help in dealing with various bacteria, fungi, and parasites etc. which cause indigestion.

Coconut oil also aids in the absorption of other nutrients, such as vitamins, minerals and amino acids. Coconut oil strengthens the immune system with its antimicrobial lipids, lauric acid, capric acid and caprylic acid which have antifungal, antibacterial and antiviral properties. Coconut oil is often preferred by athletes and body builders and by those who are dieting, to other oils, as its fat content is easily converted into energy, does not lead to accumulation of fat in the heart and arteries and boosts athletic performance.

Kelp contains the complete spectrum of minerals needed by man, as are contained in the ocean itself. Kelp granules are especially rich in potassium, iron, iodine, Vitamin B-6, Riboflavin, and dietary fiber. Even more important than the minerals needed in relatively large amounts, such as calcium, iron, phosphorus, potassium, and so forth, are the trace minerals- iodine, copper, manganese, boron, zinc, etc. These minerals appear in minute quantities in food. Our bodies need only microscopically small amounts of them.

One of the most important trace elements in kelp is iodine. This mineral is essential for the proper functioning of the thyroid which manufactures the hormone thyroxin. If an adequate amount of iodine is not provided in the diet, the thyroid gland is forced to work overtime and becomes enlarged in order to make up for the deficiency. This enlargement is known as goiter.

Phytochemicals in Kelp have been shown to absorb and eliminate radioactive elements and heavy metal contaminants from bodies. The abundant iodine in sea veggies helps to prevent the body from taking up radioactive iodine. Alginates, fucoidan and other compounds, especially in brown sea veggies like kelp, alaria, bladder wrack and rockweed, can bind to radionuclides and help our bodies excrete them. Since Fukushima, New Zealand and the North Sea are the best sources for kelp.

Lucuma powder comes mostly from the temperate Peruvian highlands, where it is stone-ground from the dried fruit of the Lucuma tree. It is similar to the egg fruit tree, in the tropics. Once known as "Gold of the Incas", the lucuma has a particularly dry pulp, which possesses a unique flavor of maple and sweet potato. Dehydrated or dried lucuma powder is a source of carbohydrates and fiber and adds nutrition to many dishes, as a thickening agent. In Peru, lucuma powder is a favorite flavor of ice cream. Lucuma can be blended into smoothies and is an excellent thickener for raw pies.

Noni is the common name for Morinda citrifolia, a tropical tree native to Polynesia, especially Tahiti and Hawaii. The fruit, leaves, stems, and roots have all been used in foods and beverages by Polynesian "Kahuna," or traditional healers, for up to 2000 years. The plant produces an irregular, lumpy, egg-shaped fruit, reaching a dozen or more centimeters in length. The ripe noni fruit and noni powder have a strong, pungent taste/odor, particularly synergistic with citrus fruits that mask the noni flavor, hence the noni species name: citrifolia.

Scientific research has identified numerous important and beneficial nutritional compounds in noni. Noni increases the efficacy of the immune system by stimulating white blood cells into "overdrive." Polysaccharide compounds found in the fruit, are believed to increase the overall power of white blood cells.

Noni fruit is also full of many powerful antioxidants and compounds to promote wellness, such as selenium (skin elasticity, skin health), xeronine (cell structure health and regeneration), glycosides (defense against free radicals), scopoletin (anti-inflammatory properties), terpine (helps the body detoxify), limonene and anthraquinones (antiseptic properties, particularly for people with compromised immune systems). Noni is a longevity superfood and immune system enhancer. In Hawaii, Noni juice is easy to make from widely available, fresh fruit.

Healthy Grains- Most people live with "gut dysbiosis" which leads to intolerance to most grains. There are four grain-like seeds that are most beneficial: millet, quinoa (keen-wah), amaranth and buckwheat. These seeds are very ancient foods used by man for thousands of years. In fact, buckwheat (not related to wheat at all) and amaranth are thought to have been cultivated 6000 years ago. They are amazing foods and are gluten-free, high in protein and in fiber.

Amaranth is an ancient grain which contains B vitamins, calcium, iron and Vitamin C. Amaranth may help lower cholesterol. Best mixed with millet/quinoa

Buckwheat is rich in flavonoids like rutin, a good source of magnesium, and is good for the cardiovascular system. It's a valuable food for those with diabetes, as it can be of help with regulating blood sugar.

Millet is an ancient grain brought to America by African slaves. It is a good source of manganese, phosphorus, and magnesium and is beneficial for the heart.

Quinoa was revered by the Incas who are said to have been the greatest agriculturists of all times. It is is a good source of iron, calcium, potassium, zinc, vitamin E, riboflavin (B2), selenium, manganese, magnesium, copper, phosphorus, and fiber! Quinoa may be helpful with migraines, diabetes or atherosclerosis. Quinoa is a quick-cooking, nutritionally dense alternative to brown rice or pasta. A ¾ C serving provides 15 grams of protein, 25 percent of daily iron and magnesium needs, and 40 percent of the daily fiber requirement. This light, delicate grain cooks in about 15 minutes or can also be sprouted. Millett is a similar delicious grain and the two are excellent cooked together.

It is always recommended to soak any grains or grain-like seeds for a minimum of 8 hours or more. Grains have phytic acid in them (as do nuts and beans) that makes them difficult to break down in the digestive system and which can bind up minerals, preventing absorption. Since most people have weak digestive systems, eating grains without soaking them could cause symptoms of digestive upset and a toxic body. Also with a healthy digestive system brown rice, especially soaked and cooked with green or brown lentils is fine in moderation.

Sprouted seeds, nuts, and grains are often referred to as live food because, in addition to being raw, they continue to grow right up to the time of consumption.

Seeds and grains contain a wonderful store of nutrients and are an excellent source of enzymes. Nature has protected the enzymes in dry seeds, nuts, grains and legumes by placing enzyme inhibitors in them. Enzyme inhibitors prevent the enzymes from being activated until the seed is germinated. Germination neutralizes the inhibitors, releases the enzymes and allowing us to receive the enzymes benefits, to aid in in the digestion of the seeds. People who have difficulty digesting seeds, nuts, grains or legumes can benefit from soaking the dry seed and beginning the germination process.
More sprouting benefits include:

1. Many seeds contain phytic acid which significantly reduces the absorption of calcium iron, zinc and other minerals, but when sprouted these losses become insignificant.
3. Nutritional value enhanced-even quadrupled.
4. Starches and sugars are converted in to simple sugars and amino acids which are readily absorbed.
5. The higher concentrations of enzymes, vitamins, minerals, amino acids, RNA etc. in sprouted foods, have a regenerative effect on the human body

For sprouting;
Use whole organic seeds, grains or nuts including alfalfa, red clover, fenugreek, radish, broccoli, mung and lentil.
For seeds, place in jar; cover and secure with a net or cloth and a rubber band. Cover with 2 to 3 times more pure water than seeds, soak overnight, for larger seeds like mung beans 16 hrs. and for smaller ones 4-6 hours.
Drain the soak water, rinse and place at a 45 degree angle, in an area with temperatures of 68-84 degrees. Rinse 2 to 3X per day through a screen till sprouts have a tail 2 to 3 x longer than the seed. Refrigerate.

Organic Fermented Rice Protein has more protein than hemp, is a low-fat, great source of energy, great supplement for athletes, also provides essential amino acids, vitamins B and E, fiber and good complex carbohydrates. Rice protein is also hypoallergenic– meaning it is easier to digest than most sources of protein.

The **Brazil nut** has the highest selenium mineral content of any food. Studies show that selenium helps the immune system and is supportive with selenium deficiencies, often found in Chron's disease and low thyroid function. Five Brazil nuts per-day is recommended.

Cayenne pepper has many therapeutic benefits including adding a spicy addition to foods, that supports "internal heat." It is an immune system stimulator as well as excellent for treating cold or flu symptoms.

Cilantro is a powerhouse of phytochemicals and a natural chelator of poisons and chemicals, like mercury and lead. It has been successfully used in cases of Autism and Alzheimer's.

Cinnamon bark is known for its delicious flavor as well as for its anti-inflammation, and sugar balancing. It is an herb used frequently in helping to stop the growth of microbial fungus/bacteria, especially Candida. Cinnamon helps people with type 2 Diabetes improve their body's response to insulin.

Ginger, along with Turmeric (Olena), are the master anti-inflammation herbs. Ginger has also been involved in numerous studies for its anti-cancer action and its immune boosting properties.

Garlic destroys viruses, lowers blood pressure and cholesterol, thins the blood, improves the release of Nitrous Oxide responsible for dilation of the blood vessels, and boosts endocrine function/sexual hormones. It is highly recommended in aiding couples in conceiving a child!

Apple pectin is excellent for colon cleansing and the apples skin & seeds have an amazing amount of beneficial phyto-chemicals. (blend well)

Basil is especially good for digestion and just about every other body system.

The inside of the broccoli stem is where the majority of phytochemicals are and is a super ingredient, when the stem peeled and blended into raw soups.

Cucumber helps to balance blood sugar by improving the body's response to insulin. The skin is also high in silica, which is the mineral for combating osteoporosis.

Pineapple is known for having the enzyme Bromelain, the majority of which is found inside the first 2 inches of the stem section, below the fruits crown leaves.

Plums are the highest known silica content food, helpful in combating osteoporosis and increasing bone density.

Raspberry seeds are the richest source of cancer fighting Ellagic acid. Blend well!

Raw apple cider vinegar contains malic acid. This chemical compound gives vinegar its sour taste and also acts as a metal detoxifier. Malic acid is well known for its ability to remove aluminum from the human body. Additional health benefits include dissolving kidney stones, relieving gout, lowering blood pressure, and balancing glucose levels.

Yacon tubers are wonderfully crisp and slightly sweet, often called "garden apples." They are mostly composed of fructooligosaccharides (an excellent probiotic food) and water which means that the majority of the carbohydrate sugars cannot be digested by the body, resulting in a very low calorie level and a prevention of excess sugar coming into the bloodstream. Yacon also helps the body increase its vitamin and mineral absorption of all other foods and is rich in potassium, calcium, and phosphorous.

Ultra-Health Adjuncts

Ayurvedic "Oil Pulling" is believed to benefit oral health in many ways. Basically, first thing in the morning, fill one tsp. with raw coconut oil or sesame oil, place in mouth and swish vigorously for 10 or more minutes. An added drop of essential oil or Olena juice is of extra benefit. When finished, discard and rinse with warm water. Search You Tube for videos of oil pulling!

Healthy Gum Drops are anti-bacterial drops which nourish the gums, teeth and saliva. This deeply penetrating formula helps nourish cells by promoting circulation to gum tissue, dentin and blood vessels within the teeth. The ingredients, individual and synergistic effects, improve and maintain gum and oral health by being a combination of antiseptic, astringent, circulatory and analgesic botanicals, promoting optimal molecular activity. Ingredients:

Tea Tree- (Melaeluca alternifolia) Clove- (Syzygium aromaticum) Rose Otto- (Rosa damascene) Cinnamon- (Cinnamomum ceylanicum) Seabuckthorn Berry- (Hippophae rhamnoides) Jojoba- (Simmondsia chinensis) Thyme Linalool (Thymus officinalis) Peppermint- (Mentha piperita) Oregano- (Origanum vulgare)

Rebounding is one of the newer forms of personal fitness and is quickly becoming popular for its affordability, effectiveness, and general appeal. Unlike normal trampolines, a rebounder is a mini-trampoline individuals use for personal fitness as well as fun. It has been associated with muscular growth, reducing arthritis pain, detoxification, quick weight loss and cardiovascular health. It is unparalleled for lymph node flushing and provides a full body workout with minimal cost, space and time.

Jumping on a rebounder can extend into many different exercises and exercise routines. Rebounding can be as simple as walking or as vigorous as a fast paced aerobic, high energy workout. A rebounder can be a money, time, and space saving decision, giving super health benefits with an amazingly short workout time, as often ten to twenty minutes per day is sufficient!

Far Infrared Sauna- Infrared rays and ultraviolet rays are invisible sun ray lights. Infrared rays are the healthiest, penetrate into the skin deeply and then dissolve harmful substances accumulated in the body. The Infrared rays vitalize cells and metabolism, and the deep heating action activates the sweat glands. Since the skin is the largest organ in the human body, the sweat glands offer one of the best means for elimination. When far infrared waves are applied to water molecules (comprising 70% of the body), these molecules begin to vibrate. This vibration reduces the ion bonds, and the eventual breakdown of water molecules causes encapsulated gases and toxic materials to be released.

Among the infrared waves, the far infrared rays, which have a wavelength of 8-14 microns, are especially good for the human body. These waves have the potential to penetrate 1.5 to 2 inches, or more, into the body allowing for deep heat and raising core body temperature from deep inside. The far infrared rays consist of similar wavelengths as those which are emitted naturally by the human body. This is one potential explanation why many people feel energetically rejuvenated and balanced from contact with far infrared waves.

Colon Hydrotherapy- When cleansing, or for general maintenance, colonics are beneficial and helpful. The colon is the central waste station of the human organism. All the waste travels through there, including residue from consumed foods, environmental toxins, chemicals and drugs. When cleansing, colon hydrotherapy is the best way to keep up with the increased waste being eliminated and to help remove impacted fecal matter on the colon walls. As the colonic removes impacted fecal matter and solid waste from the colon, what is coming out can be seen through a viewing window. In addition to solid waste, many tiny bubbles can be seen leaving the body as unnaturally oversized cells contract, shrink, and begin to pour out gaseous waste.

Inversion Therapy, also known as anti-gravity therapy, is a natural and fun way to increase circulation, relieve back pain and reduce tension and stress. Inversion has been used for thousands of years to help remove toxins, increase oxygen to cells and the brain, reduce stress and anxiety, increase energy, improve lymphatic drainage and as an effective treatment for a list of spine and back conditions. When inverted, the body and spine decompresses, providing less stress on joints, bones and muscles. Inversion can provide a "perfect" stretch and help to align the weight bearing skeleton.

Shower filter- Filtering shower tap water, especially hot water, is an absolute must on any Longevity Program. The skin readily absorbs chlorine, as do the lungs, with steam from a hot shower. A good filter will remove total chlorine, in addition to removing hydrogen sulfide ("rotten egg" smell"), iron oxides (rust water), dirt, sediment and odors for a whole year for a very low cost.

Water Filtering System- Berky water filter systems are extraordinarily effective while being very economically priced. All Berkey Water Filter systems are classified as water purifiers. In order to meet purification standards a water filter must be able to remove specified contaminants to a predetermined level, known as a "standard". This purification standard is the highest level of water contamination removal that a water filter can obtain and very few manufacturers are able to make the purification claim without the use of harsh chemicals like iodine or chlorine. Berkey does not use chemicals, instead they rely on simple, time tested, micro-filtration and a unique ionic absorption technology to purify the water for excellent results. Contact David@Berkeywaterhawaii.com 808-3736919

Excalibur Dehydrator 3000 Deluxe Series- The 3900 Deluxe Series is a 9-Tray food dehydrator, which is great for people who love healthy eating! It offers the ultimate versatility, dependability and quality construction Excalibur Food Dehydrators are known for. This Dehydrator series is designed to last over 20 years and built to the highest specifications, with upgraded components and innovative plastics. For the money and ease of use, Excalibur is the best dehydrator. 9 - 15 x 15 trays- Size 12 1/2" H X 17 W x 19 D15 square feet of drying area with an adjustable thermostat, 85 -155 degrees.

Omega FoodPro, Premier Food Processor model FP660- We have found this excellent food processor to be well made, with a functional design to make it much easier to assemble and open than many others. Stylish brushed-steel-look base, smooth wipe-clean pad and dishwasher safe parts make cleanup easy. Stainless steel two-sided shredding and slicing disks with both 2mm and 4mm capabilities; Large 11 cup work bowl handles the biggest of batches; Compact 4 cup mini-chopper is convenient for everyday tasks. Powerful, ultra-quiet, direct drive induction motor provides smooth, efficient performance and long life.

High speed Blender like Blendex, Vita mix or the economical Ninja. Single serving Bullets (with great recipes) offer speed and super easy cleaning.

Earthing Shoes etc.- These shoes allow a connection to the Earth while wearing footwear. With this practice the body becomes suffused with negatively charged free electrons abundantly present on the surface of the earth. By putting a body (positively charged) against the ground (earth) which is negatively charged, the smaller of the two will pull electrons from the larger object. The electrical potential of the two will then equalize or harmonize.

Walking barefoot on the earth (sandy beaches are great), swimming in the ocean /rivers/lakes, sleeping on a grounding pad, typing with feet on a grounding mat or walking, wearing grounded shoes can all have great health benefits. Benefits include inflammation relief, sleep improvement, blood pressure-flow improvement, lessoning of hormonal symptoms, increase healing speed, jetlag reduction, protection against EMFs from electronic devices, wireless connections, microwaves and cell phone towers. See www.pluggz.com

~~~~

"There comes a time in the life of every caring, sensitive person-a time to realize that fame is as ashes, massed fortune mere dust. It may be the last thought you think in this life. If at such a time you can truly say, "I have done my best," and your only regret is that you could not have done more, then you will have done very well indeed."
-Dynamic Harmlessness, H J Dinshah, Powerful Vegan Messages

~~~~

Kirtan chanting and meditation provides access to quieter, more balanced parts of the Self. Through Kirtan chanting and meditation access and relationship is gained with all parts of our being. The mind becomes quieter, our awareness is expanded and we balance our being. Many Kirtan chants have been sung for thousands of years and carry the momentum and blessings of the Holy Beings who have resonated with these chants. This is a powerful practice to invoke and invite Divine help, align the chakras and dispel barriers to our true self.
The "Maha Mrityunjaya Mantra" is one of the most powerful chants/mantras of all, having been chanted down through the ages by countless spiritual masters and disciples. A favorite, it is of particular benefit in longevity enhancement, as it is known as the protector and curer from diseases, the "Death Defying Mantra."

Om Tryambicum Yajamahe- We meditate on the three eyed one, Lord Shiva
Sugandhim Pushti Vardhanam- Which permeates and nourishes all like a fragrance
Urvarukamiva Bandhanan- May we be liberated from death for the sake of Immortality
Mrityoor Mukshiya Mamritat- Even as the cucumber is released from its bondage to the vine.

90

For a powerful rendition, I was blessed to be part of recording, along with more super mantras, check out *Karunamayi –"Power of Chant" on CD Baby* downloads www.cdbaby.com/cd/karunamayi

Some favorite Kirtan artists are Deva Premal and Mitten, Krishna Das, Shantalla, Brenda McMorrow, Jaya Lakshmi and Ananda….

~~~~

"Our experience of pain for the world springs from our inter-connectedness with all beings, from which also arises our powers to act on their behalf. When we deny or repress our pain for the world, or treat it as a private pathology, our power to take part in the healing of the world is diminished."
-www.Joannamacy.net

Skillful Lifestyle Practices - 300 points

____Vegan, organic, plant based diet (25)
____Gluten free (5)
____Super food breakfast (10)
____Regularly consume cultured vegetables (5)
____Shop at farmers markets (5)
____Drink ½ body weight, in oz.'s, of clean, filtered or spring water daily (10)
____Make and consume own coconut water Kefir or Kombucha (5)
____Have a large glass of fresh vegetable juice 3+ times/week (5)
____Have a home garden (5)
____No GMO, hydrogenated, rancid or canola oils. (5)
____70-30 to all raw diet (10)
____Supplement with concentrated superfoods (10)
____Use digestive/protolytic enzymes (5)
____Probiotics (5)
____Antioxidants: Apothe Cherry, Astaxanthin (5)
____Vegan EFA oils- Phytoplankton, hemp, borage, etc. oils (5)
____Immune boosting and anti-fungal herb formulas (5)
____Focused, long term cleansing program, 1x year (20)
____Participate in a cleansing retreat, at a center, 1 week/year (20)
____Knowledge of and basic use of Ayurvedic and Chinese Tonic herbs (5)
____Minimal VOCs (Volatile Organic Compounds) - See Detoxification chapter (5)
____Minimal EMFs, (Electro Magnetic Frequencies) (5)
____A ten minute, or more, meditation practice daily (5)
____Devotional singing practice (5)
____Have a community of likeminded, health oriented, friends (20)
____Study spiritual growth/Wisdom Tradition teachings (20)
____Say a blessing/gratitude prayer before eating (5)
____Watch supportive media input regularly (5)

___Exercise 3+ times/week for ½ hr. or more (10)
___Spend some time in nature weekly (5)
___Walk barefoot on earth 20+ minutes, 3 or more times / week (5)
___Receive bodywork (Acupuncture, massage, etc.) at least 2 times/month (5)
___Colonics' a few times/year (5)
___Far infrared sauna 2+ times per month (5)
___Use a shower water filter (10)
___Organic and clean body care/sun block oral care (5)
___Safe household cleaners (5)
___Organic chemical free yard care (5)
___? 300 total points, possible

Pillars of Ultra Health and Longevity
For a longer, more active and fulfilling life!

- A organic whole foods/superfoods diet that is nutritionally dense, plant strong mostly raw, low glycemic, gluten free, food-combined and balanced, as low on the food chain as possible with appropriate supplementation.
- Exercise, inversion, rebounding, swimming
- Deep sleep - balanced hormones, brain chemistry
- Colonics/massage, bodywork, far infrared sauna
- Chemical free body-care, dental care, and cleaning products
- Healthy water (spring, low mineral) without plastic containers and installing a shower filter to remove chlorine.
- Living and working free of VOCs (Volatile Organic Compounds) and excessive electrical fields (EMFs)
- Mercury amalgam removal and heavy metal detoxification.
- Time in nature, barefoot on the Earth, grounding, yoga, exercise.

A thorough cleanse- comprehensive 1- 3 month detoxification and rejuvenation program which alleviates the root causes of most inflammation, gut disturbances, ill health - including mental, while counteracting many of the main aging factors.

Longevity Source Cleanse Overview
Main points and options, with the 80-20 diet

If facing a health challenge, or "health opportunity" in Optimum Health Institute rephrasing, we highly recommend one of the detoxification centers listed in the Resources section and/or finding an Integrative/Functional Medicine Doctor.

The Longevity Source cleanse (LSC) is a long term cleanse meant to be thorough yet gentle, life changing, yet at a pace that is easy to manage. Options are given when to integrate each phase and increase quantities.

Many of the health products are from Purium Health Foods. We have found all these ultra-pure, high vibration, organic, GMO free, concentrated superfood/herb formulations to be extraordinarily effective in supporting health and longevity. We have also found Purium health products to be of the highest quality, the company unparalleled in its business practices, model and educational mission. Purium owner, David Sandoval's book "*The Green Foods Bible*" is exceptionally informative for detailing the core principles and sources of health and wellness!

~~~~

"Within weeks, a diet rich in vegetables, fruit and concentrated green "superfoods" will reduce inflammation, improve elimination, and reduce oxidation's toll on the body. Some green foods will speed the elimination of toxins from the body and protect against the DNA damage and oxidation they can foster. They'll boost the intake of enzymes and alkalinize the body. We can lose weight which in turn will lower the risk of many chronic illnesses."
Purium founder, David Sandoval- *The Green Foods Bible*

~~~~

As we comfortably settle into the LSC (Longevity Source Cleanse) protocol, it's then much easier to add another ingredient or change amounts! Please be gentle and honor personal situations! All ingredients purpose and qualities are listed in the *Longevity Source* book with dietary supporting, excellent bulk superfood sources found online through the *Longevity Source* website, Resources section.

~~~~

"Valuing the sacredness of food means eating soulfully, which in turn implies that particular attention is given to what we choose to take from outside to nourish the inside. Most of our culture, physical and social, operates as if there was no interior life, or at least assumes that the interior life has little or nothing to do with the outside world. Retrieving the sacred in our lives demands that we bring back enchantment into everyday actions and processes.

Enchantment in our surroundings for instance can be found if we begin to think in terms of having a house (and planet) for our bodies, a home for our hearts and a temple for our souls. The building, the place where we live remains the same, but under the spell of enchantment it is perceived as nurturing three very different, albeit equally important functions.

The same enchantment can be brought back to cooking and eating. These can be seen as the two magical functions of nourishing and healing our bodies. The kitchen then becomes a temple where, magically, food is alchemically transformed into a glorious substance that sustains us in all dimensions."
-Mascetti and Borthwick, Food for the Spirit

Cleanse Design and Objectives

The Longevity Source Cleanse is designed to give maximum results by targeting specific, common, areas of toxin buildup and optimal bodily function disruptions.

1. Removal of toxins and chemicals from cell wall membranes and any layer of fat coating cell walls, to improve cellular hydration.

2. Supplying optimal nutrition that supports increased oxygen and glucose (glycogen) availability and uptake, for increased cellular energy (ATP).

3. Supply bio-available nutrient support for the methylation process to effectively release xenoestrogens and other endocrine disruptors (pesticides, herbicides fallates from plastics, etc.), from the liver and other receptor sites.

4. The chelation and excretion of any heavy metals (arsenic, mercury, lead etc.).

5. Dissolve calcium deposits and pathogen produced, "bio-shields."
6. Strengthen the gut biome and immune system, repairing any "leaky gut" issues while cleansing and strengthening colon walls.

7. Curtail overpopulations of Candida yeast, fungus, virus, molds, pathogenic and opportunistic organisms.

8. Build muscle mass while eliminating stored fat.

9. Supply the targeted nutritional support of full spectrum melatonin while removing common areas of calcification, including the pineal gland.

10. Reset metabolism and dietary habits with optimal nutrition foods.

All the previous are intentionally designed with the objective of helping transform the lifestyle and direction of our lives, to lengthen Telomeres, and to turn on good genes while turning off unbeneficial ones. This can then help maximise longevity, health and fulfillment of life purpose, and in so doing help to transform the planet!

~~~~

"I have devoted nearly two decades of my life to discovering foods that heal and making them available in their purest possible, non-crossbred, wildcrafted forms. The foods that I seek are designed by nature and especially easy to use and assimilate. The thousands of lives I have been able to improve and the renewed hope that people feel is the fruit of those efforts, and my pride and joy."
-D. Sandoval, The Green Foods Bible, Purium Health Products

Core Cleanse Ingredients
(may substitute with similar formulas available online or in HF store)

Ionic Elements is an all-natural, mineral rich, dietary supplement with the highest possible concentration of pure ocean trace minerals, activated with Fulvic acid. PHP's Ionic Elements have no preservatives and yet naturally will stay potent over time.

Fulvic Acid is extremely valuable in its action as a chelator of unwanted calcium deposits and as a protector against toxic heavy metals. It even improves brain function. Fulvic acid acts as a "free-radical" scavenger, supplies vital electrolytes, enhances and transports nutrients, catalyzes enzyme reactions, increases assimilation, stimulates metabolism, chelates and changes inorganic minerals into organically complex minerals. It modifies the damage of toxic compounds such as heavy metals and free radicals and increases the permeability of digestive, circulatory and cell membranes, to help detoxify.

Supercharged activated fulvic acid with ocean and plant derived magnesium and over 72 Ionic trace minerals. This mineral-rich dietary supplement was specially formulated to help support and maintain a healthy immune system, promote increased hydration and circulation, with a boost in natural energy and vitality.

Zeolites are a deeply detoxifying, and alkalizing group of volcanic minerals that support a powerful, natural chelating process. When taken orally they allow the release of harmful toxins and heavy metals from the body. Formed eons ago by the interaction of volcanic lava with ocean waters, zeolites have a unique molecular structure resembling a honeycomb or cage-like design. The lattices of the zeolite cages hold a natural negative charge which attracts and irreversibly binds positively-charged toxins. It's the main, safe for human consumption, remedy for radiation, mercury, and pesticide toxin exposures.

The importance of a smaller particle size is it yields a considerably greater overall zeolite surface area. This allows a significantly greater number of "cages" to be exposed, thereby increasing the ability to absorb toxins and heavy metals. This formulation is enhanced with organic preservative-free aloe vera, ionic ocean minerals and minimal amounts of concentrated fulvic acid, which support the chelating potency and help naturally preserve the liquid zeolites.

Purium's Power of 10 Veggies is a synergistic combination of green foods and herbs that have been used for centuries to fight the signs of aging. It's recommended to use this product with Purium's Apothe-Cherry for the best defense against aging. Helps protect against cellular oxidative stress. May help increase energy and vigor. May support healthy cardiovascular function and healthy immune function. Purium's "More Greens" (which is similar and has probiotics) may be used in place of Power of 10, or use Power of 10 in the AM and More Greens in PM. Instructions:
Mix ½ scoop with 8-10 oz. of cold water or juice and drink daily. Works best when taken on an empty stomach.

Ingredients: Ho Shu Wu, Cat's Claw, Amla, Astaxanthin, Aloe Vera 200:1, White American Ginseng, Organic Barley grass whole powder, Organic Oat grass whole powder, Organic Spinach, Organic Broccoli, Organic Kale, Organic Parsley, Organic Spirulina, Organic Chlorella, Organic Dandelion Leaf, Organic Cilantro, Organic Dulse, Organic Wheat grass whole powder, Organic Alfalfa grass Juice Powder, Organic Arabic Gum, Lo Han Guo berry Extract, Organic Apple Flavor, Organic Raspberry Flavor.

Purium More Greens- Spirulina, Oatgrass juice powder, Organic Alfalfa, Kamut, Wheat grass whole leaf powder, Organic Barley Grass juice powder, Arabino galactin, Rice Bran Solubles, Inulin-FOS, Carrot Juice Powder, Bee Pollen, Pineapple natural flavor, Cruciferous vegetable blend- Broccoli, Cabbage, Kale and Parsley powder, American Ginseng, shelf stable probiotic blend, Chlorozyme, cracked cell Chlorella, Kelp, Broccoli Sprout, Lo Han Guo

Super Lytes- Contains Rooibos tea extract for rapid rehydration. Also contains quality sodium from Himalayan sea salt, balanced with added magnesium and potassium to reduce cramping and headaches.

Super CleansR is a unique combination of herbs & superfoods that enhances deep cleansing by stimulating peristaltic action and elimination gently and effectively. Contains ingredients that have been shown to defend the body from parasites.
Black Walnut Hull, Marshmallow, Clove, Wormwood, Amalaki, Cascara sargata, Senna Leaf

Daily Fiber Blend is unlike any other fiber product on the market. It is designed so that the body gets the purest and most potent protein, essential fatty acids, enzymes, and essential fibers for comprehensive digestive and immune support. May enhance bowel function while supporting healthy cardiovascular function and a weight loss regimen. Contains highly digestible amino acids.
Servings per container: 30. Excellent combined with Super CleanseR

Instructions: Take 1 scoop (2 tbsp.) mixed with water, juice, or your favorite smoothie- best taken 1-2 hours before bedtime or instead of a snack.

Ingredients: Flax Seed, Acacia Gum, Rice Bran, Psyllium Husk, Apple Fiber, Activated Barley, Chia Seed , Inulin - FOS (Fructooligosaccharides), Fennel Seed, Glucomannan (Amorphopallus konjac), Black Walnut, Pineapple Powder Flavor, Sprouted Quinoa, Sprouted Amaranth, Sprouted Spelt, Sprouted Kamut

Apothe-Cherry- The known benefits of cherries continues to increase. According to ongoing research, Montmorency tart cherries are a rich source of antioxidants, which can help fight cancer and heart disease. In addition, there are beneficial compounds in Montmorency tart cherries that help relieve the pain of arthritis and gout. Other fruits and vegetables do not have the pain relief of tart cherries. While the research on the exact mechanisms that give the pain relief is ongoing, many consumers are discovering that tart cherry juice and other cherry products can stave off pain. Research also shows that tart cherries are a rich source of powerful antioxidants, including kaempferol, quercetin and melatonin. Melatonin is a powerful antioxidant considered more potent than vitamins C, E, and A, because cherry juice concentrate, which involves greatly reducing the water content, has ten times the melatonin of the raw fruit.

Produced in the pineal gland at the base of the brain, melatonin controls sleepiness at night, wakefulness in daytime and functions as an antioxidant to help the body destroy free radicals. Melatonin is also an excellent remover of bad estrogen from the liver. There are about 100 fresh cherries in a one ounce glass of this cherry juice. Apothe-Cherry is a pure Montmorency tart cherry liquid concentrate that mixes with juice or water.

Tart cherry's capacity for scavenging free radicals, identified as its "ORAC," in each serving of Apothe-Cherry is more than 7,000 units. This is comparable to the ORAC levels of raspberries. Instructions: 1 Tablespoon in water at bedtime.

(40x) Aloe Vera- Aloe is one of the most revered of all African herbs and has been exported to every corner of the world. Hippocrates himself called aloe "the potted physician" for its amazing healing properties. We recommend combining it with Purium's Apothe-Cherry. Supports healthy immune function, may aid in healthy digestion, supports healthy joint function and healthy blood glucose levels. ½ tsp. in water, morning and evening.

Master Amino Complex- A pre-digested, 100% vegan protein that has been featured extensively in the Physician's Desk Reference and is a non-soy, totally assimilable protein source, with no binders, fillers, or excipients. The ultimate protein, MAP is our name for the patented, clinically proven "Master Amino Acid Pattern" (MAP) created by Dr. Luca Moretti.

Ingredients: Patented proprietary blend of non-soy legumes, 5,000 mg:
L-Leucine L-Valine, L-Isoleucine, L-Phenylalanine, L-Threonine, L-Methionine L-Tryptophan, L-Lysine

Use Master Amino Complex, together with a balanced diet, to aid in normalizing protein synthesis, assistance with the stabilization or recovery of muscle strength, endurance and volume and for help keeping body tissues firm, with minimization of body fat. Master Aminos may also be helpful for weight loss, for children and adults suffering from ADD and for improvement in the quality of life.

Astaxanthin- Super Xanthin (as ZAN thin) is made from nature's most powerful antioxidant, When it comes to free radical scavenging, Astaxanthin can be as much as 65 times more powerful than vitamin C and 54 times stronger than beta-carotene. Astaxanthin is even potentially so effective, it's able to cross the blood-brain barrier and protect the brain and nervous system from oxidative stress!
It helps combat free radical damage to muscles and helps reduce the buildup of lactic acid that causes post-workout soreness. May enhance metabolism, support eye health and improve recovery time while protecting muscle tissue from damage. It can also provide some protection for the skin from UVA and UVB damage. Instructions:
Take two capsules a day. When exercising, it is best to take one before beginning a workout and one after. Best to take with a meal or source of good fat. Ingredients: Haematococcus Microalgae; Spirulina, Cellulose capsule.

C from Nature is a natural, powerful combination of Indian Amalaki, Acerola, Camu Camu, rose hips, and citrus bioflavonoids that is unsurpassed by any synthetic or manufactured vitamin C product. Because of the proven health benefits of vitamin C, we recommend taking this product with Fulvic Zeolite™ for detoxification.
Contains powerful anti-oxidants and ingredients that promote the rapid absorption of vitamin C. May support healthy immune function, promote healthy cholesterol levels and cardiovascular function, promote increased serotonin levels. Instructions:
Have 2 each with morning and evening Longevity drink
Ingredients: Amla Powder (Embilica ocinalis), fruit; Acerola Extract, fruit; Camu Camu Extract, fruit; Citrus Bioavenoids; Rosehips (Rosa canina)

Renew Hair, Skin, and Nails is a unique and effective natural plant and herb blend that provides targeted nutritional support to help the body rebuild specific collagen from the inside out. It's recommended to combine this product with Power of 10 Veggies to support optimal health for hair, skin, and nails.

Helps strengthen hair, nails, and skin and may help prevent split ends and breakage. Promotes healthy, younger-looking skin. May support natural stress relief. Ingredients may act synergistically with Fulvic acid and Zeolite
Instructions: Take 1 (or more) capsules, each with morning and evening Longevity drink.

Ingredients: Spirulina, Ho Shu Wu, Lignisul MSM (Methyl-sulfonylmethane), Horsetail, Bamboo Extract, Organic silica, Dandelion, Saw Palmetto, Kelp, Ginger Root Rhizome, Grape Seed Extract (ActiVin®), Lutein

Vir-U-Sure is a proprietary blend of herbs and whole foods that offer synergistic, targeted support for healthy immune function and viral response. May support natural healing processes. Virusure contains sulphated polysaccharide compounds that support a healthy immune response to viruses.
Instructions: Take 1 capsule, each with morning and evening drink and up to 6 capsules daily for more therapeutic support.

Ingredients: Red Algae Gigartina, Red Algae Dumontacea, Neem Extract Bitters (Azadirachta indica), Olive Leaf Oleuropein (Oleae europaea), Spirulina (Spirulina platensis), Oregano Oil Powder (Origanum vulgare), AES, Assimilating Enhancing System - Aspergillus based enzymes and trace minerals

Advanced Probiotic Blend is a potent, all-vegetarian blend of the most vital, friendly bacteria available. We recommend supporting the body's immune system by taking Purium's Advanced Probiotic Blend™ in conjunction with any of our green foods. It is dairy-free and does not need to be refrigerated. Supports healthy levels of good bacteria, aids in healthy digestion and can help improve nutrient absorption while supporting healthy immune function.
Instructions: Take one capsule each with breakfast and lunch.
Ingredients: Proprietary Blend: L. gasseri, B. bifidum, B. longum, L. paracasei; Lactospore (B. coagulans); Inulin-FOS (Fructooligosaccharide); Fiber Gum (Acacia); cellulose capsules.

Enzyme Advantage is a patented, shelf-stable, aspergillus derived formula that helps the body break down and assimilate nutrients in the foods we eat. This also ensures that no food remains in the body undigested, causing gastrointestinal distress or discomfort. We recommend combining this product with Advanced Probiotic™ for the best digestive health. May support healthy digestion. Can help eliminate toxins, may support healthy immune function and may enhance nutrient absorption when taken with meals. May also be used as part of a natural allergy defense regimen. Instructions: Take two capsules (or more) with cooked dinners.
Ingredients: Protease, Lipase, Amylase, Cellulase, Calcium, Magnesium, Zinc, Manganese, 72 trace minerals, and sea kelp

LOVE Supermeal- Live, Organic, Vegan Energy in a glass! L.O.V.E. contains 12 green foods, 10 vegetables, 9 sprouts and 5 mushrooms! L.O.V.E. is non-GMO, gluten-free, soy-free, and dairy-free! Each of the 36 ingredients is 100% certified organic and 100% vegan. L.O.V.E. Super Meal is 7 products in 1! Weight Loss Formula, Protein Drink, Fiber Supplement, EFA Supplement, Super Antioxidant Drink, Immune Support Supplement, Energy Drink

Ingredients: Organic Fermented Rice Protein, Organic Flax Seed, Organic Green Food Blend *(containing Alfalfa Leaf Juice Powder, Wheat Grass, Barley Grass, Spirulina, Chlorella, Dandelion Leaf)*, Organic Sprout Blend *(containing: Quinoa Sprout, Red Clover Sprout, Sunflower Sprout, Flax Sprout, Amaranth Sprout, Lentil Sprout, Millet Sprout, Garbanzo Bean Sprout, Broccoli Sprout)*, Organic Dark Buckwheat, Organic Mushroom Blend *(containing: Maitake, Cordyceps, Tremella, Shitake, Turkey Tail)*, Organic Maca, Organic Pumpkin, Organic Vegetable Blend *(containing: Broccoli, Cabbage, Parsley, Kale)*, Organic Apple Extract, Organic Rhodiola Root, Organic Eleuthero Root, Organic Acerola Cherry, Organic Stevia Extract, Organic Sea Kelp and Dulse.

Power Shake- The Power Shake was created so that one could easily consume several "power foods" (that have ancient roots as potent fuels for energizing the human body) all-at-once, thus saving time and money. When combined, these whole foods help the body have long term sustained energy, endurance, and strength. They also provide protection from catabolic damage. Ingredients:

Activated Barley*: Research demonstrates that the best energy source for the body is a slow-burning carbohydrate that provides well-balanced blood sugar and insulin levels. Purium's patented, natural method of pre-sprouting activates the nutrients and enzymes in the inner kernel of the barley pearl increasing its energy potential by 400% and increasing the beta glucan content by up to 94%, over traditional barley grain products.

Organic Carrot Juice Plus*: Known as one of the most important parts of any juice fast or raw food regimen, it's deep, rich, orange color comes from the abundance of beta-carotene, minerals, and other phyto-nutrients that are unique to the tuber family.

***Organic Kamut Blend*:** (Kamut wheatgrass, oat grass juice, and alfalfa leaf juice) The use of wheatgrass has moved from healing clinics to juice bars due to its phenomenal effect on the body. Its high nutrient content makes it great for detoxification, for aiding the digestion system, and naturally increasing energy.

Rice Bran Solubles*: Scientific studies indicated that Rice Bran Solubles are vital for maintaining normal cholesterol levels and blood glucose control. They are also an all-natural source of vitamin E type tocopherols and tocotreinols and contain a variety of B vitamins, co-Q10, gamma oryzanol, folic acid, and more.

Hawaiian Spirulina: Nature's most complete nutrient source, containing over 60% complete vegetarian protein, an abundance of chlorophyll and essential fatty acids, vitamins, minerals, and nucleic acids, as well as nature's highest source of a new class of immune enhancers, a photosynthetic pigment called phyco-can.
Combined Potential Benefits:
A readily available daily vitamin and mineral source with other nutrients needed for a proper diet. Helps balance blood glucose levels, improves digestion, assimilation, elimination and circulation. Provides an immune system boost. Mix 1 slightly rounded scoop with 10-20 oz. of water or freshly prepared green vegetable juice. Take on an empty stomach, 2 times per day between meals.

Women's Defense- Maitake, Reishi, Shiitake, Lion's Mane, Agaricus, Cordyceps, Turkey Tail, Tremella, Sprouted Soy (Glycine Max); Cat's Claw Extract 4:1 (Uncaria tomentosa), Bark; Red Clover Extract 40% Isoflavone (Trifolium pratense), Flowering tops; Fermented Soy (Glycine Max); GliSODin™

Purification Practice
Taking refuge in the Three Jewels- the Buddha, the dharma and the sanga

"To take refuge in the Buddha is to take refuge in someone who let go of holding back, just as we can do. To take refuge in the dharma is to take refuge in all the teachings that encourage and nurture our inherent ability to let go of holding back. And to take refuge in the sanga is to take refuge in the community of people who share this longing to let go and open rather than shield themselves. Fundamentally even though other people can give us support, we do it ourselves, and that's how we grow up in this process, rather than becoming more dependent." -Start Where You Are, A Guide to Compassionate Living,
-Pema Chodron

Mindfulness Training

"Aware of the suffering caused by un-mindful consumption, I am committed to cultivate good health, both physical and mental for myself, my family and my society by practicing mindful eating, drinking and consuming. I am committed to ingest only items that preserve peace, wellbeing and joy in my consciousness..."
-Thich Nhat Hahn, Going Home, Jesus and Buddha as Brothers

~~~~

Longevity Source Cleanse Protocol
with Purium Health Products and dietary shifts!

<u>Zero</u>- Processed foods, GMOs, high fructose corn syrup, gluten, casein, coffee, non-plant based foods.

Minimize- (After 10 Day Transformation Cleanse)- Sweet/dried fruits, organic gluten free breads, organic potato chips, corn chips, rice cakes/chips, bean chips/crackers etc. (Raw dehydrated crackers are great!)
Minimize caffeine! (including green tea, mate, chocolate/cacao...)

Integrate- An organic wholefoods, plant based, low glycemic diet. Add coconut water kefir and sauerkraut, green juices, smoothies, with about a 70-30 raw to cooked diet (outline follows). Drink 2-3 quarts of clean/purified water per day. (1.5 quarts before breakfast, and 1 quart before lunch, is a good start!)
Total cost for recommended cleanse is les than $100 per week for 12 weeks. There can be a significant saving on food costs, as less food is needed, and processed foods are eliminated. The 10 Day Transformational Cleanse and Weight Loss Pack provides exceptional results by giving 3000 calories worth of nutrition with only 600 calories of concentrated superfoods. It also includes; the gentle, deep and effective cleansing properties of the Super CleanseR, the replenishing and rehydrating of the Super Lytes, muscle mass improvement and fat burning stimulation of the Master Amino Protein and high melatonin and ORAC content of the Apothe Cherry, all adding up to a truly effective cleanse and life-changing-enhancing program. (Also, one or more colonics will benefit greatly)

For those wishing to maintain weight, or have an easier start, during the 10 day cleanse, a suggested "Flex Food" menu is included at end of this section. For adrenal and energy support, Puriums Bee Energetic is extraordinarily effective. Feel free to adjust timing with your own flow!

For the most economical cleanse version, begin with a 10 Day Transformational Cleanse then continue with the basic protocol of Power of 10 Vegies, (or More Greens or Chlorella powder), mixed with water, lemon and Zeolite drops for the morning and evening drink. (Include daily use of LOVE Meal or Power Shake, with a whole foods diet for best results!)

The 10 day Transformational Cleanse guidelines are outlined in the Purium Transformation Guide (available at www.mypurium.com/vegancheftodd- gift card) and Superfood Chef Todd's version 1.5, which follows LS cleanse.

~~~~

"Old habits are broken, not by self-coercion, but by attraction to new habits that give an awakened sense of aliveness" -D. Sandoval

Longevity Source Cleanse, for the first four weeks (30days)

(After the first 10 day Transformation); begin with 3 bottles of regular LOVE Meal.
1 Power of 10 Vegies, 1 More Greens, 1 Renew Hair, Skin and Nails, and
1 bottle Apothe-Cherry.
Also add 1 bottle Ionic Elements and 1 bottle Chlorella tablets
Opt. To this add, if needed, the digestion relief booster pack (40X Aloe concentrate, Enzyme Advantage*, Advanced Probiotic blend)* and Daily Fiber blend. (The fiber is well suited to add to the 10 Day Cleanse) Asterisk= optional.

AM- 8-12 oz.'s pure water with ½ serving (scoop) of Power of 10 Veggies, with a squeeze of lemon/citrus and 5 drops Ionic elements. (Ginger, Olena punch in Recipes section is an excellent base!) Opt. ½ tsp aloe concentrate,* 5 to 10 drops Kyolic aged garlic extract.

Take 1 capsule Renew Hair Skin and Nails with drink.
If practicing oil pulling, follow pulling with drink.

Before breakfast have 1 Advanced Probiotic Blend,* if needed.
Breakfast (after finishing the 10 Day Transformational Cleanse)
1 scoop each Purium LOVE meal and More Greens. Add 10 chlorella tablets, fruit, berries and soaked seeds, in the Magical Morning LOVE Breakfast (beginning of Recipe section).

Mid-morning- 1 scoop LOVE meal with coconut water or fresh seed/nut milk, and 10 drops Ionic elements.
Opt. make a double breakfast and have 2nd breakfast.
In drinking water add 5-10 drops Ionic elements per quart. Consume a minimum of two to three quarts per-day, of pure water.
Mostly raw lunch with added sauerkraut and 1 cap, Advanced Probiotic Blend.*
(See Meal Planning Ideas to follow.)

Afternoon- ½ serving (2 scoops) LOVE meal in freshly made green/red vegetable juice, coconut water Kefir, or water.

Plant-based dinner with sauerkraut, as outlined next, with 2 Enzyme Advantage.*
PM (well after dinner)- ½ to 1 C water, citrus, ½ tsp Aloe concentrate,*
1 T Apothe Cherry, ½ scoop Power of 10 vegies, 5 drops Ionic elements and 1 capsule Renew Hair Skin and Nails.

For the second 4 weeks

Continue, as previously, by resupplying 1- 30 serving LOVE Meal pack (adjust to personal consumption). Add a Power of 10 Vegies and More Greens. Also add one bottle each Virasure, C from Nature (250), Fulvic Zeolite and Super Xanthin. For morning and evening drink use Fulvic Zeolite (Replacing Ionic Elements), starting with one drop per drink and ½ serving of Power of 10, then build to three to four drops per drink, over a week or two.

With both morning and evening drink, add taking two capsules C from Nature and 3 Virasure (More if needed for Candida etc. symptoms). Add 1 Super Xanthin each, before breakfast and dinner or before and after exercise.

For the last 4 weeks

Resupply- 1 LOVE Meal Continuation Pack.
Continue previous month's protocol to finish all supplies!
Continue to improve dietary and lifestyle habits as appropriate.

~~~~

"The Yoga Sutras speak of the mind in the first chapter, and the body in the second chapter and they remind us in the third chapter and fourth chapters that our final aim in Yoga must be to arrive at the soul. Yet within the science of Yoga the three levels of being-body, mind and soul-are all involved. Thus Yoga is an integrated science which can lead mans divided being back to wholeness and health." -BKS Iyengar, TheTree of Yoga

~~~~

"Spirituality is a commitment to live deeply enough within yourself to be present to what is happening now and open to what the next step is. It does not require the final step, only the readiness for the next one, and the next. That is how I became a spiritual practitioner and how I became a vegetarian. The next step, that is your spiritual path." -Carol J. Adams, The Inner Art of Vegetarianism

10 Day Transformational Cleanse, Version 1.5
For an easier start or weight retention!

7 am– 5 MAPs & 1 Super Lytes, water, slices of apple, starfruit, grapefruit
8:30– Smoothie with fruit bowls;
2 Bowls- ½ apple and ½ pear chopped and ½ C blueberries evenly divided
Blend- ½ C soaked sunflower seeds and ½ apple and ½ pear and ½ C blueberries, ½ of an avocado and water. (Opt. coconut oil, Olena, cinnamon)

Divide between 2 bowls. Add 1-2 scoops Power Shake, 1 scoop LOVE Meal and 5-10 chlorella tabs per/bowl. Mix, when ready to eat. Save second bowl for snack
10- 5 MAPs & 1 Super Lytes, water
11:30- Second fruit bowl/smoothie and 2 capsules Super Cleanse R
1:00 pm- Vegie smoothie and salad & sauerkraut;
Smoothie- ½ cucumber, ½ zucchini, ½ avocado, kale/spinach, fresh herbs (cilantro, parsley, oregano, thyme, green onion etc.) a small beet and radish. Add water, some sauerkraut juice, lemon juice, Pink Himalayan salt, blend.
Salad- lettuce, salad greens, sprouts, grated radish, cucumber, sauerkraut. Use some vegie smoothie for salad dressing & save some for a dinner salad
2:30– 5 MAPs & 1 Super Lytes, water
4:00– 1-2 scoops Power Shake & 1 scoop fiber mix, 2 Super CleanseR
5:30– Green drink, either coconut water (fresh or in cartons, not cans) or fresh juice (cucumber, celery, green apple, beet, kale.) with 1 serving Power of 10 Vegies or More Greens. 1+ caps of Bee Energetic* may be emptied into drink to!
7:00- Steamed greens & veggies & squash: kale, broccoli, cauliflower, green beans, zucchini & kabocha squash etc. lightly steamed then add coconut oil & garlic/cayenne.Opt. Salad with sauerkraut. Vegetables with the soup…
8:30-9 pm– 1 serving Apothe Cherry

~~~~

"You can't hear it. But when you start softening and all of that gunk comes out, you really can hear your heart. As that gunk slowly releases, your heart - the arteries get cleaned out, the arteries are also lightening and softening so everything is becoming softer, more open. When that is happening, not only do you just feel better but, because you feel so much better, of course you are experiencing more love, but you are able to hear your heart." -Alicia Silverstone, The Kind Life

Food Shopping List

Farmers Market Basics
lettuce, carrots, beets, tomato, peppers, cucumber, radish, celery, cilantro, parsley, dill, basil, thyme, oregano, etc.
green onion, garlic, ginger, turmeric (olena)
zucchini, kale, cabbage, cauliflower, broccoli, green beans
starches- sweet & red potato, yam, pumpkin squash, plantain, ulu, taro
lemon, lime, grapefruit, tangelo etc.
papaya, banana, fresh berries, avocado, yacon,

Health Food Store (All the above plus);
fresh vegetables, sprouts
sunflower, pumpkin, flax, chia seeds

walnuts, brazil nuts, cashew, macadamia nuts, coconut
cacao, maca, goji berries, seeds
quinoa, millet, amaranth, brown rice, buckwheat
gluten/corn free tortillas– Food for Life, (also FFL tempeh)
red and brown lentils, mung beans, black beans, kelp noodles
sprouting seeds (alfalfa, radish, mung etc.)
sesame, olive, coconut, hemp oil, olives
raw apple cider vinegar
bulk spices/seasonings including, curry, Italian, taco, Cajun, chili, pumpkin pie, cinnamon, ginger, cardamom, etc.
miso, nutritional yeast, bulk teas
fresh fruit- apples, pears, citrus etc. dried fruit-figs, raisins etc.
fresh, dehydrated or frozen berries
PHC salt etc.
A wide selection of superfoods and supplements are available online with significant discounts (20-50%) @ Longevity Source website *Resources*!

~~~~

"We do have a choice in how we live. When we consume whole, organic plant foods, we make the best possible choice for our own personal health. When one contemplates the magnificent web of life, it comes as no surprise that what most brilliantly sustains human health will also prove ethically justifiable and ecologically sustainable.

Making healthful choices may seem like a daunting task in light of the consumer-oriented world in which we live. Rest assured that every time you have the strength and courage to make a truly conscious decision, you make this world a better place." -John Robbins

Getting Started- Choosing the 80-20 Diet

With the multitude of dietary options available, body type guidelines, changing states of health etc. it can be a daunting task for each individual to find their perfect, most healthy diet. Certain guidelines are pretty universal though, including choosing organic, plant strong, as fresh as possible (farmers markets are exceptional), gluten free, low glycemic, and for most, as raw as is feasible. We have found that the approximately 70-30 to 80-20 raw to cooked diet is ideal and can be extraordinarily healthy, especially when combined with the nutritional and cleansing protocols outlined in *Longevity Source*.

It makes sense for our lifestyle and tastes to have a simple cooked food dinner (with digestive enzymes as needed) as part of a balanced, cleansing and rejuvenating diet. Lightly cooked meals, properly food combined, often taste extra great when consuming mostly raw foods/superfoods and are easily digested and assimilated. Many people have found they can easily transition at the perfect time to even more raw foods from this diet style.

Quite a few health conscious people have found the simple Hippocrates type diet, first pioneered by Ann Wigmore, consisting of 100% raw with lots of living foods, mostly green vegetable juicing and wheatgrass juice, to work miracles! In the 1970s she had a phenomenal success rate with this diet reversing terminal cancer in the elderly at her Hippocrates Institute in Boston.

We have found the foundational recipes to be the most optimal way to begin, when exploring the 80-20 diet. I often make enough of the main dishes to last 3 or 4 days. (Salads, pates, raw soups, steamed vegetables, grains etc.) each of which take only 15-20 or so minutes to prepare. I make one or two per day, time permitting, so there is overlap, or find two main days a week (Wed - Sunday) to stock up (See Meal Planning Ideas, next).

With tasty condiments, seed sauces and garnishes, like sauerkraut or the ultra-delicious Sundried Tomato Olive Tapenade, a simple meal becomes a delightfully warming dance of flavors and textures. With occasionally dining out (looking out for GMOs) and purchasing some deli items at the health food store, it becomes a simple matter to have a healthy and satisfying diet with minimal preparation time! By shopping at farmers markets, preparing most of our own foods and foregoing nutrient deficient, calorie rich, processed, junk foods, surprisingly economical food expenses are also readily attainable.

~~~~

"We ingest excitotoxins and have no clue what those are and what they really do. We get these excitotoxins in various forms through artificial sweeteners and MSG. These artificial sweeteners are wed with artificial stimulants and made into diet drinks. We talk on radioactive phones. We eat garbage food while we watch garbage television. Our meat, fish and poultry have been exposed to such incredible amounts of poisoning and disease creating circumstances."
-Robyn Boyd, Rawsome Recipes

Meal Planning ideas

Breakfast– Magical Morning L.O.V.E. Meal breakfast, or similar

Lunch– make enough for 2-3 days- Pates', salads, kale salad, raw soups/vegetable smoothies, sauerkrauts, seed and nut butters, raw crackers, condiments. Quinoa, millet or brown rice, cooked with lentils etc. or grain alone or cooked lentils (Dahl). For snacks, on the go, make some extra morning smoothie and for lunches on the go, a gluten free wrap with grain/lentils and salad, or a salad with pate, sauerkraut, avocado, dressing along with raw vegetable soup, dehydrated crackers, Semi-raw Humus…

Dinner- prepare enough for 2 to 3 days- Quinoa/millet, plain or cooked with lentils. Steamed vegetables with steamed red potato, yam, sweet potato, squash, or, one of the "Rottin Tootin" soups in Recipe section.

Reheat only enough for the meal. For reheating vegetables, starches and grains water sauté with a little coconut oil and added fresh or dried spices and blends like; cumin, caraway, brown mustard seeds, taco, chili, Cajun, curry, Mediterranean, fresh ginger, Olena, garlic, fresh cilantro, green onions, dill, etc. For a packed meal for later, add pre-cooked vegetables, grain, soups, spices and coconut oil to a glass Pyrex dish with a fitted lid. Keep cool, when ready add hot/ boiling water and stir!

Condiments: fresh lemon juice, sesame, olive, hemp oil etc., pink crystal salt, spice blends, cayenne pepper, crushed red pepper, kelp granules, nut. yeast.

~~~~

"Wherever I go in the world, if I go to a veggie café, I am instantly tapped in to the nicest, coolest people in the town. I could be in Lithuania and think, where am I going to eat in Lithuania? And then I will find this little veggie café and all this amazing music and artists and really thoughtful, interesting people are gathering there. So it is really this beautiful way of connecting people all over the world."
-Alicia Silverstone, The Kind Life

Weekly Food Preparation, Examples

<u>Sunday</u>- Pot of quinoa/millet/ (with red lentils or lentils cooked separately) Steamed vegetables and starches, green/red juice

<u>Monday</u>- Raw seed and nut veggie pate, Kale salad
2 quarts tea (1 tulsi blend, one mineral/immune blend, for soup, breakfast etc.)

<u>Tuesday</u>- Large garden salad, Raw veggie soup/ One Island Dressing

<u>Wednesday</u>- Steamed vegetables and steamed starches, Green/red juice

<u>Thursday</u>- Pot of brown rice/brown lentils, 1 quart, Lime-Olena Gingerade

<u>Friday</u>- Large green garden vegetable salad, "Rootin Tootin" soup

<u>Saturday</u>- 1 quart jar of mung sprouts, shop at farmers market

~~~~

"The diet which serves us best will be one which produces health, limits disease, is capable of being grown and produced by natural methods, and produces enough food for all the peoples of the world."
-Janice Gray Kolb, Compassion for All Creatures

Simplified Food Preparation

<u>2x per week</u>
Raw veggie soup or one soup and one, One Island dressing
Garden salad
Seed and nut veggie pate and/or Semi-raw humus
Pot of grains with lentils or with lentils separate (dahl)
Pot of steamed veggies/starches
Opt. Green/red veggie juice

<u>1x per week</u>
2 quarts herb tea and 1 quart Lime-Olena Gingerade
1 quart sprouts (mung bean or brown lentil)
Kale salad, Pot of "Rootin Tootin" soup

<u>Recipe Abbreviations- quantities etc.</u>
C = Cup= 8 fluid ounces
tsp. = teaspoon = 3 tsp. = 1 Tablespoon
T= Tablespoon, 2 Tablespoons = 1 ounce = 1/8 C
PHC salt = Pink Himalayan Crystal Salt

"I will not continue to eat other animals," and making that choice and standing up and saying, "No!" was so profound for me as a female and as a person. It was so powerful to claim my choice and live by my beliefs and from there, to be rewarded. It was like I was rewarded with good karma because suddenly I lost all this weight, my skin cleared up, I just got so much better health. I had so much more energy. I had this lightness of feeling and so I always think of the animals as having saved me." -Alicia Silverstone, The Kind Life

~~~~

"The Unhealthy Truth is both the story of how one brave woman chose to take on the system and a call to action that shows how each of us can do our part and keep our own families safe. Robin O'Brien turns to accredited research conducted in Europe that confirms the toxicity of America's food supply, and investigates the relationship between Big Food and Big Money that has ensured that the United States is one of the only developed countries in the world to allow hidden toxins in our food—toxins that are increasingly being blamed for the alarming recent increases in allergies, A.D.H.D., cancer, and asthma among our children." www.Robynobrien.com

Foundational Recipes

Magical Morning L.O.V.E. Breakfast (for 2)
¼ C sunflower seeds & ¼ C pumpkin seeds & 1T chia seeds soaked overnight
Opt., Nuts; A few Brazil, almond, mac nut, walnut, and pecan or… Soak all overnight
Fruit: 1 green apple, 1 pear, and 2 small bananas, chopped
½ C berries
Opt. ½ avocado, 1/6 of a semi-mature coconuts pulp (healthy fat, low glycemic)
In a blender add banana-(avocado) and berries, half chopped fruit and the soaked seeds-drained with;
2T shelled hemp seeds
½ tsp. chopped ginger and/or ½ tsp. chopped fresh Olena- turmeric
Opt. 2 tsp. Maca (or to taste)
Add 1C Super Mineral Immune Boost or Tulsi/Mamaki Tea and 2 C water (or coconut water) To make about 5 blended Cups. Add any other superfoods (to taste) including Acai, cacao, Lucuma, Amla….

In 2 bowls evenly add:
Other half of chopped fruit and the soaked nuts
1T goji berries per bowl, 1 heaping tsp. cacao nibs per bowl,
Opt.1 dried fig/apricot/prune, chopped
More options; 10 chlorella tablets/bowl, some papaya, peach, lillikoi, yacon, pineapple, chico sapote, cherimoya, egg fruit …
When ready, run blender until well mixed, then pour over fruit in bowls.
Add 1-2 scoops Purium LOVE Meal and 1 scoop Power Shake, and/or other favorite Supergreen blend/ protein powder
Opt. 2 tsp. fresh ground (using a coffee grinder) golden flax seed per bowl and ¼ to ½ tsp. cinnamon powder per bowl.
Stir and Enjoy! Any extra may be kept aside for morning or afternoon snack!
For low glycemic/Candida diets, if appropriate, use low glycemic fruits like green apple, yacon, berries, avocado, raw coconut etc.

Opulent Garden Salad (enough for 3-4 meals for 2)
In a medium bowl add:
1 large head lettuce (or mix of smaller lettuces) rinsed in filtered water, drained and finely chopped
Add about 1/3 the volume of the lettuce with mixed salad greens
2 large carrots, washed, grated
1 cucumber, chopped
1 medium red pepper, chopped
2 or 3 red radishes, finely chopped/grated
Chopped fresh green onion, cilantro, parsley, baby kale

On top- 3 medium tomatoes, chopped, sprouts, sunflower, mung/lentil bean..
For festive occasions an artistic (Mandala) design can be created on top of the salad using colorful vegetables like finely chopped purple cabbage, grated carrot, red bell pepper slices, grated beets and edible flowers.

Marinated Kale and Radish Salad
½ lb. kale, de-stemmed, finely chopped
2 T olive or sesame oil
1 C finely chopped radish (pink striped radish is a colorful addition)
¼ C lime or lemon juice
1 T dried, or fresh oregano, thyme, rosemary, marjoram combo
1 tsp. PHC salt
4 cloves garlic, finely grated
Opt. 2-3 stalks green onion, finely chopped
Thoroughly mix in a bowl, by rubbing–kneading, which will shrink kale volume.
Will keep up to 4 days, in a sealed container, in fridge.

Mouthwatering Raw Vegetable Soup (2-4 servings)
1 cucumber, chopped
1 med. zucchini, chopped
1 handful, young kale, de-stemmed, chopped
¼ bunch each, cilantro, green onion and parsley, chopped
½ medium avocado
1 medium radish, chopped
1 small red beet, peeled, chopped
Opt. 2 medium tomatoes, chopped, 1-2 peeled broccoli stems, chopped
½ C soaked seeds or nuts, some semi-mature coconut pulp
Add to blender with:
1 C Mineral Immune Boost or Tonic Herb tea
2 C coconut water or water
Juice of 1-2 medium lemons or lime and/or 2 T sauerkraut juice
½ tsp. PHC salt
2 cloves garlic and or 1" Olena, peeled, chopped
Spices to your liking, (Indian, Mediterranean, Mexican, herbs etc.)
Blend on high for 1 minute.
Makes about 5 C = 2 bowls and store rest for later in fridge, (lasts 3-4 days)
Delectable as is, or serve with sauerkraut, kelp noodles, grated zucchini, mung/sunflower sprouts, avocado chunks, chopped red pepper, etc.

Sprouted Seed and Nut Vegetable Pate
1 C pumpkin and 1 C sunflower seeds and ½ C Brazil, walnut or macadamia nuts, soaked overnight or 6 hours minimum.
2 T olive, sunflower or sesame seed oil

Chopped vegetables;
1 medium zucchini
2 small red radishes
4 stalks green onion
¼ bunch each parsley and cilantro
1 medium red pepper
Juice of 1-2 medium lemons
Opt. 2 medium carrots, washed, a few kale leaves, de-stemmed, chopped
1 tsp. PHC salt
2 tsp. Mediterranean spice or 2 tsp. curry spice blend (we recommend a fresh-ground cumin and brown mustard seed mix added to fresh, finely grated turmeric (or dehydrated fresh Olena powder) combination.
2 cloves garlic, grated, a pinch of cayenne pepper, 2 Tbs. sauerkraut juice.
Food process till well mixed, stopping and hand mixing every so often.
Serve on raw crackers, in lettuce leaves, or roll up in sushi - nori sheets to make nori rolls or add to a roll with avocado, sauerkraut etc.

Living Red/Green Raw Juice
6-8 large stalks celery
2 medium cucumbers
4 medium carrots
½ bunch parsley
½ bunch cilantro
Some fresh ginger, turmeric (Olena), garlic, handful of kale, spinach, sprouts,
1 green apple
For red juice add 1 medium beet, peeled
Wash and chop all veggies for juicing, about 2 full servings = 24 or so oz.'s

Ultra Longevity Tonic Herb Tea, Concentrate
Add into a quart mason jar, 2 tulsi tea bags (or 8-12 flowering stalks from your own plant) with 1 inch peeled and finely grated fresh ginger.
Empty two capsules of Great Adaptor tonic herb formula and/or 1 bag Spring Dragon tea into jar.
Fill with boiling hot, filtered water. Cover and let steep 10 minutes, Drain into another jar and re-steep tea ingredients with first jar filled halfway with boiling water. Let stand another 10 minutes. Remove tea bags or strain loose tea.
Cover and keep in fridge. To each cup of tea add 4-8 oz. fresh water and warm for a super tonic herb tea, or use diluted for a morning tonic herbal drink, breakfast smoothie or raw soups!
Tulsi tea will turn bright red when a squeeze of lemon juice is added to tea.
Opt. Add to brew 1 T rooibos loose tea or 1 tea bag, 1 T ground shatavari root, 2 to 4 T crumbled, dried Mamaki leaves.

<u>The Super Mineral, Immune Boost Tea</u>
In a quart mason jar add 1 bag each (or heaping teaspoons of loose)
Nettles, Horsetail, Una de Gato, and Pau de Arco herb teas
Cover with boiling water, attach lid and let stand till fully cooled
Remove bags or strain tea and use for morning smoothie, in raw soups or tonic cacao drinks. Adding Mamaki leaves (Hawaiian nettles), 1/8 tsp. Chaga mushroom powder and/or 1 tsp. Ho Shu Wu powder, or adding all the above is super potent to! May be steeped a second time.

<u>Cultured Coconut Water Kefir</u>- Kefir may be made multiple ways including with raw or packaged coconut water and with added fresh juices and berries. Also, excellent Kefir can be made with either Kefir grains or with BED Kefir starter. We like the simplicity of the Body Ecology Diet product, Kefir starter (see Resource section) and have had outstanding results with it. With the BED Kefir, when once started, a portion or portions of each batch is then used to make the next batch for seven generations, as elaborated upon below:

<u>Basics</u>
30oz raw or packaged coconut water, slightly warmed to 90 degrees and added into a quart jar.
Add 1 package BED Kefir starter
Add 1 scoop BED Eco Bloom prebiotic (probiotic food) or 1 heaping tsp. coconut sugar, or favorite sweetener and/or our favorite, adding a small handful of raisins. Tighten lid, lightly shake, mixing powder well.
Stand jar on kitchen counter for 48 hrs.
After 48 hours, unscrew lid and test for fizz. If lid is overly tight, gingerly tap lid edge with handle side of a butter knife (very helpful sometimes!) till pressure release is heard. Keep tightly sealed in fridge. Lasts about seven days when regularly opened and much longer if left sealed.

From this point there are many options. At any time ¼ C or so may be taken out and added to another quart jar with coconut water and sweetener/probiotic food. Will last approximately seven generations, so making two or more new mixes at a time and leaving one unopened from each batch, till needed, will extend generations! Also when making a new mix, ½ C of coconut water may be substituted with ½ cup of Acai juice or similar. Added sweeteners for probiotic food are unnecessary when using sweet juices. Enjoy many creative possibilities!

<u>Raw Cultured Vegetables</u>
For an exotic live-zing taste sensation! This process allows for the proliferation of lactobacilli (healthful micro-flora that are naturally present in vegetables and also in our digestive tract and our compost), which break down the sugars and starches found in the vegetables, aiding the pancreas and intestines in proper

digestion. The difference between Raw Cultured Vegetables and commercially available heated sauerkrauts is the raw product is alive, 5,500,000 lactobacillus in a serving verses NONE.

Get Cultured with Donna Maltz- Culturing Your Own Vegetables, Simple Steps

Shred or cut the chosen veggies. Commonly, cabbage, beets, carrots, radish etc. In a large NON metal bowl, use your hands to kneed the veggies until the natural water from the vegetables begins to surface. At this time you can add celery juice or lemon or lime juice if you wish. I like to use a few table spoons of juice from an already fermented batch as an inoculant in each new quart I make. Some people like to add some kind of inoculants starter culture such as kefir grains, or commercial starter powder.

Add spices, herbs- garlic, ginger, Olena, cumin, cilantro etc. As the vegetable cells are broken down the mixture will notably reduce in size in the bowl and you will be ready to pack the vegetable into a wide-mouthed canning jar. The idea is to get all the air out of the jar and be sure the liquid from your mixture is covering all the veggies… This is KEY

Top with a cabbage leaf, tucking it down the sides. Again….Make sure the veggies are completely covered with juice. Loosely cover the jars, be sure they are not air tight unless you are excited about your jars blowing up. Leave at least 2 inches of room on the top as the fermentation process expands the contents in the jar.

Store in a warm, slightly moist place for 3-7 days, depending on the 4 T's; Timing Temperature Texture and Taste. Ideal temperature range is 68-75 degrees. When done, store in the refrigerator to slow down the fermentation process Option's for using less salt: If you have high blood pressure or just choose to reduce your salt intake you can do the following; Juice some celery. This is used as the brine, as it contains natural sodium and keeps the vegetables anaerobic. This eliminates the need for as much sea salt, which prevents growth of pathogenic bacteria. Fresh lemon or lime juice can be used depending on flavor preference.

Last but not least, resist the temptation to eat out of the jar, as organisms from your mouth can be introduced into the jar this way.

Tips for Making Fermented Vegetables
1 pound of vegetables = approx. 1 pint
Salts should be approx. 2-3 % of the mix about 1 tsp per pint. Ferment for 3 to 7 days at room temperature. If using an inoculant from older ferments, or a starter the process will go faster.

Timing, temperature, texture and taste, like fine wine they become even more delicious with time. Fermented Vegetable Recipe Ideas;

Colorful Kraut
3 heads green cabbage, shredded, 2 beets and 3 carrots, grated
6 TB grated ginger & 4TB fresh turmeric
4-6 TB Hawaiian or Himalayan Sea Salt
Optional: ½ lemon or lime juiced

Caraway Cumin Kraut
4 heads green cabbage shredded, or other vegetables
3 TB caraway seed, 2 TB cumin seed, 4-6 TB Hawaiian or Himalayan Sea Salt,
Optional: ½ lemon or lime juiced

Donna maltz-www.culinaryhealingartsretreat.com www.yourchoicetochange.com
Sources- Wild Fermentation- Sandor Katz www.wildfementation.com
Body Ecology- Donna Gates www.bodyecology.com
Nourishing Traditions- Sally Fallon, www.nourishedkitchen.com

Dehydrated, Raw, Flax-Vegetable Crackers
Makes about 24 cups, enough for 8 dehydrator trays.
2.5 C gold flax seeds soaked 6 hours in a half gallon jar filled with water, stir and
mix occasionally (fills jar, to make 8 cups)
8 C mixed seeds, pumpkin, sunflower etc. soaked for 4-6 hours
(makes about 10 C processed seeds)
6 C processed vegetables equals about:
4 medium zucchinis
4 chopped carrots
4 red radishes
2 medium beets
½ lb. kale, de-stemmed
2 medium peppers
Combination of fresh herbs and green onion
(Parsley cilantro, oregano, marjoram, rosemary or spiced with Indian or Cajun
seasoning mix etc.
Opt. 2 tsp. PHC salt
In a food processor add chopped vegetables and process together, then pour
into a large mixing bowl. Process some of the soaked flax with some of the
soaked seed mix, until all is processed. Mix all ingredients in a large bowl
Spread 3 C evenly per teflex sheet covered tray, making 8 trays.

Place in dehydrator and set at 140 degrees for 4 hours. Crackers will not go over
110 degrees, in this beginning stage, because of high moisture content.
After 4 hours: remove a tray and cover with the extra tray, fitted only with screen.
Holding the 2 trays tightly together flip and remove top tray and teflex sheet.

Score, now exposed soft side of cracker batter, to desired cracker size, by drawing lines with plastic knife, spatulas or Excalibur tool.

Dehydrate at 105 -110 degrees for 12-16 more hours until totally dry. Separate into individual crackers and store in sealed mason jars (add any leftover moisture absorbing packs, if available) or in a sealed container in fridge. Basically 24 C @ 3 C per tray = 8 trays and 20 crackers/tray. Ratios of 33% soaked flax, 25% vegies and 40% soaked seeds and nuts are simple basic guidelines to creatively explore with many different ratio/ingredient options.

Delicious Superfood, Cacao Fudge Pudding! (For 2 or more)
In a mixing bowl add the following:
¼ C shelled hemp seeds
¼ C Brazil nut protein powder or hemp protein powder
1 T Lucuma powder or coconut flour
2 T coconut sugar or a little stevia to taste
1-2 T cacao powder
1 T each carob powder and cacao nibs
1 T maca powder
¼ C coconut oil
Add enough acai juice or cashew milk or sunflower-coconut milk, to make pudding. Flavoring additions can include 1T fresh grated ginger, 1 tsp. cinnamon, ½ tsp. cardamom, ½ tsp. vanilla extract powder, 1 tsp. dehydrated Olena powder, 1-2 tsp. Maqui or Acai berry powders.
Optional added ingredients;
2 scoops LOVE meal, ¼ C goji and/or blueberries/ mulberries, ¼ C ground black sesame seeds, 1T chia seeds, 1 tsp. chaga powder or other favorite tonic herb powder or drops to taste! (Ashwaganda, Shatavari, Mucuna Puriens, Guduchi, Vidari kanda, Ho Shu Wu, mushroom mycelium mixes, Allow some time for ingredients to absorb moisture. Refrigerate for a thicker consistency.

~~~~

"Health is most effectively promoted by the healthful-consuming of a diet consisting of whole natural foods, exercising, getting appropriate rest, and avoiding toxic substances. Such a lifestyle not only prevents disease, but in many cases, is able to reverse disease and help restore health and well-being."
-Douglas L Lislie, Ph.D. (TrueNorth), Alan Goldhammer, D.C., The Pleasure Trap

More Recipes

Recipes are designed to be delicious on their own, or as an ideal base for creative enhancement, with one's own personal inspiration and tastes. Have Fun!

Salad and Dressing Recipes

Beet n' Carrot Salad
2 medium beets, peeled and grated
4 medium carrots, peeled and grated
1" ginger, peeled, finely grated = 2T
2 T sesame oil
2 T lemon juice or apple cider vinegar
¼ tsp. PHC salt
Opt. Add a sprinkling of soaked sunflower seeds, and or a few soaked raisins/
cranberries. Add some grated daikon radish and finely chopped yacon/cilantro.

Lentil Salad
2 C sprouted brown lentils, mung beans or mix of both
1 C chopped tomato
½ C chopped cucumbers
¼ C chopped celery
½ C chopped yellow pepper
½ C sprouts (alfalfa, red clover)
Opt. ½ C finely chopped radish
Add all vegetables to a salad bowl and serve with Island Dressing.
For sprouting mung and brown lentils, soak ¾ C beans, for 16 hours, in a quart
jar filled with water (long enough to insure all will sprout). Drain, rinse twice daily,
ready in 2-3 days. Will fill jar when sprouted and sprout tail is length of seed.

Island Dressing- (blend all)
1 C chopped tomatoes
½ C cashews, soaked 1 hour
¼ C oil (sesame, olive, sunflower)
¼ C lemon juice
¼ C raisins or dates
1 med. cucumber, chopped
¼ C chopped red pepper
¼ C chopped green onion
¼ C chopped cilantro
2 tsp. cumin powder
Salt to taste- about ½ tsp. PHC salt

Avocado Veggie Salad (Romaine wraps)
1 large avocado, seed and skin removed
1 yellow beet, peeled and grated
2 red radishes, grated
1 medium zucchini grated

½ bunch cilantro, finely chopped
2 garlic cloves, finely grated
2 limes, juiced and/or 1 T sauerkraut juice
Opt. Some chopped yacon, pinch of cayenne pepper to taste
PHC salt to taste
Mix well! For Romaine wraps add a couple spoonful's, lengthwise to a Romaine lettuce leaf with Opt. added sauerkraut, seed pate, roll up lengthwise and enjoy!

One Island, Avocado Herb Dressing- blended
1 C water, coconut water or Longevity Tulsi tea
½ medium avocado
1 large broccoli stem, peeled, chopped
1 peeled beet
½ med. zucchini, chopped
½ C fresh coconut pulp (if available)
1 lemon, juiced and 1 T sauerkraut juice
1-2 T chopped, fresh garden herbs (cilantro, parsley, thyme, oregano etc.)
2 cloves garlic, minced
½ tsp. Hawaiian sea salt

Pink Tahini Dressing or Sauce/dip- (blended)
½ C raw tahini
½ C filtered water
2 tsp. freshly squeezed lemon juice
2 T finely chopped green onion
2 tsp. raw apple cider vinegar
1 tsp. garlic/ginger, minced
½ tsp. PHC salt or 1 tsp Sea Clear or chickpea miso, to start
A pinch of cayenne and/or cumin powder
Blend in a medium sweet red pepper and/or ¼ C soaked, sun-dried tomatoes to add a beautiful pink color. Opt. Blend-in two pitted medjul dates.

Sun-dried Tomato Pesto- Blended
½ C water
¼ C olive oil
½-1 C chopped fresh basil & ¼ C chopped parsley
¼ C Sun-dried tomatoes, soaked 1 hour
¼ C lime juice
2 T chopped green onion
4 cloves garlic, chopped
Opt. 2 medjul dates, pitted, ½ C soaked seeds/nuts
1-2 tsp. White Miso
Blend/process well

Marinara Sauce
1 C chopped tomato
½ C sun-dried tomatoes, soaked ½ hr. in water
½ red bell pepper, chopped
2 T shredded beets
1 T olive oil
1 T nutritional yeast
1 T dried basil
1 tsp. each dried oregano and thyme
2 cloves garlic, finely chopped or grated
½ tsp. PHC salt and cayenne pepper to taste
Process to smooth consistency.

Nut and Seed Butter
1 C sunflower seeds
1 C pumpkin seeds
½ C Brazil or macadamia nuts
Opt. ½ C shelled hemp seeds,
2 T sesame oil and 2 T coconut oil
PHC salt to taste (start with ½ tsp.)
Process well, stir occasionally, and then process more to a smooth consistency.
Add more oil if needed. Experiment with combinations of nuts, seeds, oils. A high
speed blender may also be used, hand stirring occasionally.
Excellent Tahini (sesame butter) can be simply made by finely grinding sesame
seeds in a coffee grinder,(opt. with sunflower seeds) then adding sesame oil to
desired consistency.

Macnut, Sunflower and Cashew, Zucchini Pate'- (process all)
2 C sunflower seeds and cashews, soaked 1-2 hrs.
½ C macadamia nuts, soaked 2-4 hrs.
2 C chopped zucchini
¼ C chopped cilantro
2 T chopped parsley
¼ C lemon juice
4 cloves garlic, chopped
4 medium green onion stalks, chopped
2 T sesame oil
2 T nutritional yeast & ½ tsp PHC salt or to taste
1 tsp. cumin seeds and 1 tsp. brown mustard seeds, freshly ground

Semi-Raw Hummus
1 can Eden garbanzo beans, drained (or 2 C of cooked)
4 T sesame seeds finely ground in coffee grinder

4-6 med. kale leaves, destemmed, chopped
1 med. zucchini, chopped
2 large cloves garlic, finely grated
1 T lemon juice and 1 T sauerkraut juice
1-2 T olive oil or sesame oil
2 tsp ground cumin and1 tsp PHC salt
Rosemary, parsley or cilantro and cayenne pepper to taste, process well.

Green Olive Tapenade or Raw Pizza Topping
In a mixing bowl add;
½ C chopped, raw olives and/or
1 C chopped bottled organic green olives
¼ C chopped walnuts (or pecans), soaked 2 hours
¼ C sun-dried tomatoes, soaked in water 20 minutes, chopped.
2 T olive oil
2 green onion stalks, finely chopped
½ bunch parsley, de-stemmed and finely chopped
1 tsp. finely chopped, fresh thyme
4 cloves garlic, finely grated
Juice of 1 medium lemon
½ tsp. PHC salt or 1 tsp. Sea Clear or Miso-Master Chickpea miso paste
May be lightly food processed for maximum flavor integration!
For raw pizza sauce, add 1 C chopped fresh tomatoes and additional ¾ C
soaked sun-dried tomatoes to the ¼ C in recipe (total of 1 C). Process well.

Mango Salsa- Chutney
3 C fresh, peeled and chopped mango
2 T sesame oil and ¼ C lime juice
3 stalks green onion, finely chopped
3 medium garlic cloves, finely grated and 1T finely grated, fresh ginger
¼ tsp. crushed red chili flakes and 1 tsp. fresh ground, brown mustard seeds
Opt. 2 T fresh chopped mint and ½ C soaked raisins, chopped
PHC salt to taste, Mix well, makes an excellent garnish or side dish!
For a cooked version add 1 C water with 1 tsp. coconut flour, lightly blend. In a
small sauce pan, bring to a light bubble, then simmer on low a couple minutes.

Raw, Vegan Tom Yum Soup (Coutesy of Under the Bodhi Tree Restaurant)
2 ½ cups coconut water, preferably raw
1 cup raw cashews
3 tbsp. coconut oil
3 tbsp. + 1 tbsp. Nama Soy Sauce (raw soy sauce)
1 leaf Kaffir lime
1 tbsp. + 1 tsp. ginger, fresh, peeled and clean

2 cloves garlic
1 Hawaiian chili pepper
½ cup shredded raw coconut
½ cup thin sliced carrots
½ cup Bok Choy, sliced thin
½ cup Shiitake mushrooms, thinly sliced
Place the shredded coconut, 1 TBLS coconut oil, kafir lime, garlic, ginger, chili pepper, and cilantro into a food processor and chop until it's a smooth paste
Add the chili paste from the food processor to the blender and blend the mix until smooth and creamy
Place the cashews, 2C coconut water, 1 TBLS coconut oil, and 3 TBLS Nama soy sauce into a vita-mix blender
Combine 1 TBLS Nama soy sauce, 1 TBLS coconut oil, 1 pinch minced garlic, and 1 pinch minced ginger to1/2 cup coconut water to make the vegetable marinade.Pour the marinade over the fresh raw veg and toss, hold in refrigeration. Place 8oz of coconut cream broth into a bowl, place 3 tbls of marinated veg mix into the soup, top with fresh cilantro.

Cultured Coconut- Macnut "Yogurt"
1 C soaked macadamia nuts (4+ hours)
1 C fresh coconut pulp (medium/semi soft to rubbery)
2 T sauerkraut juice and enough coconut water (2 C) or water to blend well
Blend, add to quart jar with lid loosely fastened, place on kitchen counter 4-8 hrs.
Move to fridge, lightly seal lid. Ready in 2-4 days with a tart and sour taste!

Raw, Vegan, Cucumber Yogurt, Raita
Mix following ingredients with 1½ C pre-made cultured coconut-macnut yogurt
1 med. cucumber, grated
½ bunch cilantro, finely chopped
2 tsp. lemon juice
1 tsp. ground cumin and 1 tsp. ground coriander powder
Opt. 1 tsp fresh mint, finely chopped, ¼ tsp crushed red chili flakes
PHC salt to taste. YUM!

~~~~

"Again, going back to the fact that not only is it the healthiest way to live (vegan), but this is also the answer to our environmental problems, to ending suffering. I am all about being efficient and effective and if you could do one thing that knocks out so many other things at the same time, it's a very good use of time. So that really excites me." -Alicia Silverstone, The Kind Life

~~~~

Dehydrated Foods

Sprouted Mung, Lentil Burger
2 C mixed, sprouted brown lentils/mung beans
1 C sunflower seeds and 1 C pumpkin seeds soaked 2-4 hrs.
½ C chopped green onion
½ C chopped red pepper
1 C chopped zucchini
1 C de-stemmed and chopped kale
6 cloves garlic, finely grated
Either, 1 T fresh ground coriander and 1 T fresh ground brown mustard seed or
1 T dried oregano and 1 T dried marjoram
2 tsp. PHC salt
¼ C freshly ground fax seeds,Opt. 2 plantains, peeled, chopped
Mix all ingredients in a bowl, add half at a time to food processor and fully
process, then mix together.
Form into patties or balls, place on teflex sheets and dehydrate at 140° for 4 hrs.,
flip onto screen and then dehydrate at 105° 12-16 more hours.
Makes about 30 patties fitting on two, 14"X14" screens/trays.

Raw Buckwheat Crackers, Patties, Cookies- base recipe
1.5 C buckwheat, soaked 4 hours, drained, soaked 2 more hours, drained
1 C sunflower seeds, soaked 4 hrs.
⅛ C flax seeds, soaked in ½ C water 4 hours

Vegetable Crackers- Pizza Crust (1 tray, about 24 crackers, or 1 raw pizza crust)
To base recipe add 1 cup chopped vegetables; like zucchini, kale, carrot and
green onion, and fresh herbs, and some spices, like Mediterranean or Indian.
(Basically, about 4 Cups equals 40% sprouted buckwheat, 10% soaked flax, 25%
soaked seeds/nuts, 25% vegetable mix)

Mix well in a food processor. Dehydrate following the flax cracker recipe,
previously shown, for dehydrating, flipping and scoring directions.
(About 4 hours at 140° then flip, score and 12-16 hours more at 110° for
complete dehydrating. For pizza crust, batter may also be formed into a round
pizza shape with triangular scoring).

Curried Vegetable Patties- Add another cup of finely chopped vegetables to
cracker recipe like zucchini, cauliflower, peppers, kale, beet. Process with 1 T
cumin powder, 2 tsp. ground mustard seeds and 1 tsp. raw turmeric, 1 tsp. PHC
salt. Form into 16 patties and dehydrate (Follow Flax Cracker recipe directions
for flipping). Patties may need a little longer to fully dehydrate. Extraordinary
served with chutney and raw raita!

Cookies- To the base recipe, add ¾ C mixed raisins, dates and, figs, soaked 1 hr. (soaking expands fruit to about 1 C) with just enough water to cover. Add 1 tsp. cinnamon and 1 tsp. nutmeg. All or half of the soaked, dried fruit mix may be reprocessed into batter, with the other half finely chopped, then mixed into already processed batter.

Opt. Add 1 medium banana, 1 inch ginger finely chopped, some cacao nibs, goji/ blue berries, ½ chopped apple etc. and process well.

Form batter (with added chopped fruit) into 16 cookies

Dehydrate same as above, flipping after 4 hours or so. Serve with cacao fudge!

Banana, Raisin, Macnut Cookies (16)

½ C sunflower seeds, soaked 4 hours
½ C macadamia nuts, soaked 4 hours
½ C pumpkin seeds, soaked 4 hours
1 C raisins soaked 1 hr., in just enough water to cover
½ C soaked and drained coconut flakes
2 medium bananas, peeled and sliced
4 T ground flax seed
1 tsp. cinnamon and ½ tsp. nutmeg and 1 T fresh ginger
Process all ingredients well.

Opt: leave out some mac-nuts, seeds and raisins, fine chop and add into processed batter.

Form into 16 cookies per teflex sheet and dehydrate at 140° for 4 hours then flip onto screen and continue dehydrating at 105° for 12 -16 more hours.

May also add chopped apple, pineapple, grated or chopped mango, more soaked coconut flakes etc. Makes 16 good size cookies= 1 tray

Savory and Crunchy Kale Chips

1 bunch (½ lb.) de-stemmed curly leaf kale, chopped into bite size pieces
2 T coconut oil and 1T lemon juice
2 T ground flax seed and 2 T nutritional yeast
1 tsp. Mediterranean, Spanish, or curry seasoning (may include fresh, finely grated garlic or Olena, or a pinch of cayenne pepper to taste).
4 T soaked sunflower seeds, plus ½ tsp. PHC salt

Process well, except kale, then add kale and mix thoroughly. Place batter covered kale leaves on dehydrator shelf. Follow standard dehydrating method!

~~~~

"That is really where I was coming from. I want people to be kind to themselves first and make themselves feel their best and not need to depend on medicine and not need all of those things I just mentioned. And also at the same time they just accidentally (by choosing vegan) are being shepherds of the Earth and for the animals and of the people who are starving." -A. Silverstone, The Kind Life

Beverages

Lime, Olena, Gingerade- (Awesome Longevity Drink base)
Juice from 2 med. juicy limes
1" (by about ½ inch) each, peeled and chopped, ginger and Olena
Pure water to fill 1 quart jar
Opt. Substitute some tonic tea, coconut water, citrus juice, for equal parts water.
Blend on high for 1 minute.
This blend excels as the base for morning and evening Longevity drink!
For an Ayurvedic rejuvinative add to 2 oz.'s Gingerade with 2 ounces water; 1/8 tsp each Mucuna and Guduchi and ½ tsp each Vidari kanda and chlorella powder. For a sparkling beverage add some Kombucha or coconut Kefir.

Fresh Noni Juice and Olena, Super Punch
Pick enough close to ripe (whitish) noni fruits to fill a 2 qt. covered jar then place jar on counter. As the fruits ripen they exude a pale liquid. Pour off liquid every day and drink as is or mix into the morning Longevity Drink.
Any extra may be stored in a sealed glass container in fridge.
For Punch; 1 large fresh ripe noni, added to blender with one cup water,
Blend till well pureed, then pour through strainer to remove seeds
Pour strained noni liquid back into blender with 1 C water, blend and use as is, or mix well with 3 C Lime-Olena, Ginger aid!

Super Berry, Zinger Lemonade
½ tsp. acai powder, contents of 1 cap Purium- C from nature
2 C water or 1 C water with 1 C coconut water or coconut water kefir, pomegranate juice, kombucha, cold tonic herb tea.
¼ C lemon juice
Opt. Add one serving of Purium, Power of 10 veggies, More Greens or chlorella!

Nut and Seed Milk
1 C nuts/seeds- macnut, cashew, sesame, sunflower (hemp) soaked 4-8 hours and drained except hemp seeds do not need to be soaked.
3.5 C water
Blend nuts and seeds with 2 C water, on high for 1 minute. (Add 1" each Olena and ginger, then blend for an extra boost)
Strain, add 1.5 C water and blend again, re-strain, save unblended bits for smoothies, cookies, desserts etc.
Sweeten nut milk to taste; coconut sugar, stevia, blended in dates etc.
Excellent in warm tea and as a cacao drink base with LOVE meal and berries.
Makes one quart (plus ½ C or so) plant strong milk.
Alternatively: If soaking ½ C seeds (pumpkin/sunflower) for use in breakfast, soak ¼ C extra. Drain, then add to blender with 1/6th of a semi-mature coconuts

(rubbery) pulp and 2 C water. Blend for 1 minute-strain for extra creamy coco-sun milk. Add 2 C more water and blended remains for original use in breakfast. (For super quick coconut milk, blend 1 package of frozen coconut milk or BPA and guar gum free can of Native Forest, organic coconut milk with equal amount water then store in a quart jar, in fridge. Shake well before each use)

Cacao, Super Tonic Cacao
1 C nut/seed/coconut milk, or similar
1 C Tonic Herb Tea base, or Mamaki/ Tulsi Tea or Spring Dragon Tea
½ tsp. Olena powder or 2 tsp. fresh root
2 tsp. finely chopped fresh ginger
1 T cacao powder and 2 tsp. carob powder
½ tsp. cinnamon, ¼ tsp. cardamom, ¼ tsp. vanilla extract
Options add:
2 tsp Maca powder, 2 tsp. Purium Apothe-Cherry (for cherry cacao), ½ tsp. Chaga mushroom powder. Add stevia or coconut sugar to taste, blend well, warm in pan. For a super Ayurvedic heart, hormone and head tonic add ¼ to ½ tsp each Arjuna, Ashwaganda and Brahmi-bacopa.

Fresh Berry-Cacao Tonic Smoothie– blended
1 C mixed, fresh or frozen raspberries, blackberries, blueberries
1 C tonic herb tea and 1 C coconut water or water
½ C cashews, soaked 1 hour
¼ C raw cacao powder
2 tsp. maca powder and 2 tsp. Lucuma powder

"There is a social myth that life without meat and dairy is difficult, prone to malnutrition, and void of satisfaction and texture. On the contrary I've found that the healthier my eating habits have become, the more flavors and culinary joys I have discovered. I am now in better physical health than I have ever been, with more stamina and zest for life." -John Robbins, The Food Revolution

Desserts

Superfood Bliss Balls
1 C sunflower seeds (or macadamia nuts etc.)
1 C raisins or figs, chopped and soaked in just enough water to cover for 1 hr.
½ C coconut flakes
¼ C coconut oil
¼ C goji berries
2 T cacao nibs
2 T shelled hemp seeds

2 T Lucuma powder
Opt. 2 T carob or cacao powder or combination
1 T cinnamon, 1 T Maca, 1 tsp. Chaga powder
Add all ingredients (including soak water) into food processor, except gojis and process well. Add to mixing bowl with gojis and combine well. Form into 1" to 1.5" diameter balls, which also may then be rolled in more coconut flakes!

Chia Seed Pudding
¼ C chia seeds
1 C sweetened liquid (nut milk with stevia or 1 C acai juice or ½ C nut milk and ½ C blueberry puree or 1 C coconut water.
Soak together till fully thickened (about 2 hrs.)

Chia (mock) Tapioca Pudding
1.5 C fresh "coconut milk" from nut/seed milk recipe or 1 C coconut water blended with ½ C soaked cashew nuts, sesame or (unsoaked) hemp seeds or combo will make a "coco-nut" milk. Then mix with ¼ C coconut flakes. Add ½ tsp. vanilla extract and ¼ C chia seeds. Add stevia or coconut sugar to sweeten.
Let stand 2+ hours, to fully thicken.

Mocha like Avocado Mousse
1 C ripe avocado
¼ C Medjul dates, pitted
4 T cacao powder and 2 T carob powder
1 tsp. cinnamon (Opt. add ½ tsp. ginger, cardamom etc.)
1 C cashews soaked 1 to 2 hrs. and/or 2 bananas
¼ C coconut oil
1T Dandy Blend or similar coffee substitute
1 tsp. cinnamon and ½ tsp. cardamom or other similar spices
Opt. 2 scoops Purium LOVE Meal
Combine in food processor, refrigerate to set.
Double this recipe to make a great raw pie filling!

Lemon Ginger Sauce
¼ C dates soaked in ½ C water (or coconut water)
½ C soaked and drained, cashews or macadamia nuts
2 T lemon juice
1 T grated ginger
Food process or blend. Use date soak water for liquid.
Excellent on raw pies, coconut ice cream, cacao pudding etc.

Hemp seed, Macnut, Blueberry Sauce- Base
½ C shelled hemp seeds

½ C macadamia nuts or cashews soaked 4 hrs.
2 T lucuma powder
1 C coconut water or water
¼ C cacao powder and ½ to 1 C blueberries
Opt. 2 tsp. Purium Apothe-Cherry
Blend to a smooth consistency.
Excellent on raw pies.

Sesame Goji (Cacao) Balls
2 C sesame and 1 C sunflower seeds, soaked 4 hours, rinsed
½ C shredded coconut
8 medjul dates, pitted, mashed
¼ C goji berries
¼ C coconut oil
¼ C lucuma powder
2 tsp. cinnamon
½ tsp. nutmeg
Opt. add, ¼ C cacao nibs, ½ tsp. cardamom
Food process thoroughly, some or all gojis can be left out and added in after processing. Form into balls or cookies and refrigerate. Will last weeks, can be frozen. For more crunch add ½ C pre-chopped macnuts to processed dough.

Basic Raw Pie Crust
1 C of nuts or seeds, or mix (macadamia nuts, almond, sunflower, pumpkin etc.)
1 C coconut flakes
½ C mashed, pitted dates
2 T raw coconut oil
2 tsp. cinnamon
Opt: 2 T cacao nibs
In a food processor mix to a sticky consistency. Add more oil if needed.
Spread evenly on a lightly oiled pie plate, pressing crust out to form edges.

Mango or Peach Pie etc.
2 C cashews or macadamia nuts soaked 2+ hours
3 C mango chunks or other fruit (peach, apricot etc.)
½ C dates, coconut sugar or other sweetener
½ C coconut oil
2T finely grated ginger, ½ tsp. cardamom Opt. 1 T lemon juice, 2 T lucuma
Mix in a food processor leaving out 1 C of the finely chopped fruit to add in after processing, spread and distribute evenly. Refrigerate to set.

Avocado, Cacao-Raspberry Pie
4 C avocado and ½ C cacao powder

½ C coconut oil
½ C pitted dates or coconut sugar
1 C soaked cashews
1 C raspberries
Opt.1 medium banana, 1 T cinnamon, 4 T raw carob powder,
2-4 scoops LOVE Meal or Power Shake or combo, 1 T Purium Apothe-Cherry
Form pie crust, using previous recipe, and set in freezer.
Add rest of ingredients to food processor and process to smooth consistency (if adding raspberries, leave out ½ C). Pour processed filling into crust (add raspberries, spreading evenly). If adding Apothe-Cherry drizzle on top.
Keep in fridge for a few hours to set.

Award Winning (Hawaii Avocado Festival)- Key Lime or Blueberry Pie
1 pie crust recipe made with macadamia nuts
2 large or 3 medium avocados,
1 C macadamia nuts soaked 2-4 hrs.
6 medium key limes, juiced and the zest of 1 lime
½ C coconut sugar
½ C coconut oil (add opt. cup of fresh coconut pulp)
2 T grated ginger
Form pie crust and set in freezer. Add rest of ingredients to food processor and process to smooth consistency. Pour into crust and set in freezer for 1-2 hours.
Opt add 1 C blueberries into puree for a delicious Blueberry Key Lime Pie!

Foundational Cooked Foods

Basic Grain-Lentil Dish
2 C grain (quinoa/millet) with 1 C red or French green lentils or
2 C brown rice with 1 C, either brown lentils, split peas or Mung Dahl
Soak overnight, drain, rinse well. (½ C amaranth may be substituted for equal amount of any of the other grains).
Instead of cooking with the normal 6.5 C water add 5 C water to soaked/drained mix, bring to boil, then cover and lower to #2. Heat until fully cooked. Soaking shortens usual cooking time by up to 1/3. Total cooking time of about 15 minutes for quinoa/millet mix and 30 to 35 minutes for rice mix. After turning off heat leave pot covered for a while to insure dish is fully cooked!

Quinoa/Rice and Vegetable Curry
3 C cooked quinoa or quinoa/lentil combo or cooked brown rice
2 C mixed, previously chopped and steamed, vegetables/starches; broccoli, cauliflower, zucchini, red pepper, green beans, chopped red potatoes, yams, sweet potatoes, Ulu, plantain..
1" finely chopped Olena and 1" finely grated ginger

1 tsp. fresh ground coriander
1 tsp. fresh ground brown mustard seeds
½ tsp. cumin seeds
¼ bunch cilantro, finely chopped
Opt. Add 3 chopped tomatoes
Add vegetables and spices (except cilantro) to a pan with ¼ C water and a little coconut oil.

Water sauté on medium heat till steaming hot.
Lower heat, add quinoa/rice, 1T coconut oil, chopped cilantro and mix well and heat to steaming hot. Mix in PHC salt or chickpea miso to taste

Kabocha Squash, Vegetable Curry
1 medium Kabocha squash baked or steamed, skin and seeds removed
2 cans (BPA free) organic coconut milk (or frozen in bags product is awesome)
2 C steamed vegetables; kale, cauliflower, green beans etc.
2 T finely grated ginger
2 T chickpea miso
1 T curry powder
½ bunch cilantro, chopped
1 lemon, juiced
Blend all ingredients except vegetables, adding some water if needed
Simmer for a few minutes, add vegetables and cilantro, turn off and let stand briefly, then serve.
Opt. add pinch of cayenne pepper, ½ C lemongrass tea, 1T grated Olena

Purple Sweet Potato or Yam- Veggie- Sunflower Seed patties
3 med. large size yams or sweet potato's peeled and 1 large red potato trimmed to fit through food processor chute with slicer attached.
½ med zucchini and 4 large kale leaves - destemmed (for sw. potato patties) or
¼ medium cauliflower head &1/2 med. zucchini (for yam patties).
Add either set of ingredients & potatoe to food processor with slicer attachment.
Process, then empty and place blade attachment in processor. Refill with either yam or potato ingredients.
Add ½ C millet flour and ½ C sunflower seeds- (finely ground in a coffee grinder) or `½ C mac-nut flour
Opt. add ½ C garbanzo flour
Add 3 generous tablespoons coconut oil and spices of choice.
1 T cinnamon, 2 T minced ginger, etc.
Opt. some fresh coconut pulp and curry powder
Process to a thick paste like texture (Add a little coconut oil if needed)

With a ¼ C measure scoop out mixture and make approx.15 patties on a standard baking dish (10x15 inch) oiled with coconut oil, or use a 1/8 C measure and make 30-40 or so mounds.
Bake for 25 minutes at 365 degrees, remove and flip, and cook for 15 more minutes.

Popoulu (Plantain) Vegetable Patties
3 large plantains, peeled and chopped (Popoulu and Mohouli are varieties of Hawaiian cooking bananas) Equals about 2.5 to 3 C when blended
1 C chopped vegetables- zucchini, kale, carrot, peeled beet etc.
1 C sprouted mung beans
1 C soaked sunflower seeds
2 T coconut oil PHC salt
1 T curry spices, or Cajun seasoning or Mediterranean spices

Mix well in blender or food processor, stopping occasionally to stir mixture
Make patties (about 12-3 inch wide) place on a coconut oiled cookie sheet
Bake at 350 degrees for 20 minutes, flip and cook for another ten minutes then shut off oven and let sit for another 20 minutes. Best vegie burger ever!
Patties also may be dehydrated instead of cooked. Adding some Ulu is yum!

Rootin Tootin Soups- creative variations
Purple sweet potato and potato with kale and ginger
Dilled potato- leek with green beans, caraway and red pepper, lemon juice
Yam and potato soup with cauliflower, cinnamon and nutmeg or curry spices
Beet, carrot, daikon and fennel with broccoli coriander and garlic (sun-dried tomato's)

Prepare about 6 medium size root vegies, mix of choice (clean, peel etc.)
Cut to size to fit through food processor slicer and slice all roots & vegies
Fine chop, garlic, ginger etc. to taste
Add to pot with Opt. 2 tsp. coconut oil, spices and salt to taste and enough water to cover. Bring to boil and simmer till cooked. (20 min.) Mash with potato masher or, when cooled, blend some or all. Cook kale in soup for last 10 minutes. Add other vegetables, steamed, after mashing, blending. Makes about six good servings! This may serve as a base for various vegetable stews with added steamed vegetables, coconut milk, tomatoes and different spicing options.

~~~~

*"**Moms in Charge** is a MOVEMENT for moms to become EMPOWERED with information of what is in our food and products so we can make the MOST informed decisions and TRANSITION to a healthier, vibrant life with our kids. Childhood obesity and diabetes are rising at an alarming rate. Cancer remains*

the number one disease that kills our kids. The majority of kids affected by the cold, flu and allergies has increased so much that they are now considered "common". OUR MISSION IS TO BE PART OF THE SOLUTION. As you become a part of this community, you will be supported and know you are not alone and you are also a part of a MOVEMENT to CHANGE THE SHAPE of our future; a future where giving our kids healthy food and products is not only accepted, but expected. I'll see you on the journey!" Momsincharge.org

Resources for Sustainable and Healthy Living

John and Ocean Robbins, www.foodrevolution.org- The Food Revolution Network is an online-based education and advocacy-driven initiative committed to healthy, sustainable, humane and conscious food for all. Guided by John and Ocean Robbins, with more than 100,000 members and with the collaboration of many of the top food revolutionary leaders of our times, the Food Revolution Network aims to empower individuals, build community, and transform food systems to support healthy people and a healthy planet.
John Robbins is an award-winning bestselling author of nine books, the founder of EarthSave International, and one of the world's leading spokes-people for healthy food for a sustainable world. John and his son Ocean are co-founders of the Food Revolution Network.

Ocean is CEO of the Food Revolution Network and co-author of, *Voices of the Food Revolution*. He has spoken in person to more than 200,000 people from 65+ nations, and serves as an internationally acclaimed speaker and facilitator.

Dean Ornish- Ornishspectrum.com Dr. Ornish's 37 years of research has scientifically proven that the integrative lifestyle changes he recommends can: improve chronic conditions – such as heart disease, diabetes and prostate cancer, change gene expression, turning on health-promoting genes and turning off disease-promoting genes, lengthen telomeres — the ends of chromosomes - which begins to reverse aging on a cellular level
For more info: www.ornishspectrum.com/proven-program

~~~~

"We pay for things that are dangerous, invasive, expensive, and largely ineffective. Stents and angioplasties don't work for stable patients, and the surgery for prostate cancer isn't really necessary most of the time. Meanwhile, the power of these very simple, low-tech, low-cost interventions like diet and lifestyle changes have become increasingly well-documented. The opportunities are really ripe now for industries to realize a new paradigm of medical care that can be much more sustainable, and even profitable." -Dean Ornish MD

~~~ ~

Jeffery Smith- Executive Director, Institute for Responsible Technology
www.Responsibletechnology.org
www.NonGMOShoppingGuide.com
Director, Genetic Roulette -The Gamble of Our Lives
www.GeneticRouletteMovie.com
International bestselling author of Seeds of Deception and Genetic Roulette
www.SeedsofDeception.com

www.Vegsource.com- At VegSource, we believe there's a lot more to vegetarianism than what you put in your mouth . . .

We believe that being a vegetarian is a good start. It's a healthier way to live physically, as well as ethically and (dare we say?) spiritually. If you can teach a child from the very beginning to be kind to animals -- the weaker links in our society -- then it's not such a huge leap that they'll grow up to be people who are kinder to human animals, as well.
We decided to bring a number of preeminent medical doctors who were all using a low-fat plant-based diet to cure people of many different diseases together into a health super forum. My wife dodged a fatal disease bullet because she was blessed to get good information. We brought these top experts together and videotaped their powerful presentations so others could get the knowledge to protect or completely restore their own health too. We recommend our documentary PROCESSED PEOPLE. It's 40 minutes long, and the DVD also contains another 2.5 hours of extended interviews where the MDs talk about a variety of subjects you'll want to hear!

Will Tuttle- www.worldpeacediet.com The World Peace Diet has been called one of the most important books of the 21st century: the foundation of a new society based on the truth of the interconnectedness of all life. Dr. Tuttle offers lectures, workshops, and trainings internationally on The World Peace Diet, veganism, spirituality, effective activism, meditation, and intuition development.

Alicia Silverstone, www.Thekindlife.com- The Kind Diet, The Kind Mama
This website is an excellent resource for those who want to delve deeper into the world of healthy, green, eco-friendly living. The Kind Life is a hub to get valuable information and find resources to help make every aspect of life as kind as possible, detailing all of the things in my life that have helped me to be as kind to the planet as possible. Let's get inspired together and help each other to live the healthiest, kindest lives possible!

www.Richroll.com What makes Rich Roll truly remarkable is that less than two years prior to his first Ultraman, he didn't even own a bike, let alone race one. Although he competed as a butterfly swimmer at Stanford University in the late

80's, Rich's career was cut short by struggles with drugs and alcohol -- an addiction that led him astray for the next decade, alienating friends, colleagues and family, landing him in jails, institutions and ultimately rehab at age 31.

Although sober, Rich soon found himself 50 pounds overweight; the furthest thing from fit. Everything came to head on the eve of his 40th birthday. Defeated by a mere flight of stairs that left him buckled over in pain, he foresaw the almost certain heart attack looming in his near future. The day immediately following his staircase epiphany, Rich overhauled his diet, became a dedicated vegan, put on his running shoes and jumped back into the pool.

It wasn't long before ambition took hold and his quest to participate in Ultraman slowly began. Two years later, 50 pounds lighter, and fueled by nothing but plants, he surprised the triathlon & ultra communities by not only becoming the first vegan to complete the 320-mile über-endurance event, but by finishing in the top 10 males (3rd fastest American) with the 2nd fastest swim split -- all despite having never previously completed even a half-ironman distance triathlon. Rich is now considered one of the worlds top ten athletes, a leading advocate for plant based diets and a vegan restaurant owner.

A Few (more) of the Real Food Movement Heroes;

Robyn O'Brien- Founder, Chief Inspiration Officer, AllergyKids Foundation
As a former food industry analyst, author and mother of four, Robyn O'Brien brings compassion, insight and detailed analysis to her role as the founder of the organization and her research into the impact that the global food system is having on the health of children.

The mission is to restore the health of our children and integrity of our food supply. The goal is simple and straightforward: we want to protect the American children from the additives now found in our food supply – additives not used in children's foods in other developed countries. In our efforts to achieve this, the AllergyKids Foundation works to:

Inspire choices that enhance the quality of life, improve nutrition and create change in the health of our children, schools and communities.
Inform parents and caregivers about food grown without the use of synthetic additives, artificial growth hormones and pesticides.

Address the increasing prevalence of synthetic additives, artificial growth hormones, antibiotics and genetically engineered allergens and proteins now found in the U.S. food supply and its impact on the health of our families.

Provide materials and resources to help individuals and families reduce their exposure to additives in their diets.
Cultivate team building and grassroots movements that drive change in our schools, communities, organizations, and food supply.-www.robynobrien.com

Vani Hari- Foodbabe.com The typical American diet landed her where that diet typically does, in a hospital. It was then, in the hospital bed more than ten years ago, that she decided to make health her number one priority. Vani used her new found inspiration for living a healthy life to drive her energy into investigating what is really in our food, how is it grown and what chemicals are used in production.

Vani Hari is now a revolutionary food activist, a New York Times bestselling author, and was named one of the "Most Influential People on The Internet" by Time Magazine in 2015. Hari started FoodBabe.com in April 2011 to spread information about what is really in the American food supply. She teaches people how to make the right purchasing decisions at the grocery store, how to live an organic lifestyle, and how to travel healthfully around the world. The success of her writing and investigative work can be seen in the way food companies react to her uncanny ability to find and expose the truth.

Tony Robbins- www.tonyrobbins.com, Keys To An Extraordinary Life.
Paul McCartney & Family- www.meatfreemondays.com, Singing and Standing for Healthy Food.
Congressman Tim Ryan- timryan.house.gov, Sane Food Policy…
Joel Furman, MD- www.drfuhrman.com, Eating for Optimal Health.
Vandana Shiva Ph.D- www.navdanya.org, Food, Democracy & the Future of Life
Francis Moore Lappe- www.smallplanet.org, How We Can End World Hunger
Will Allen- www.growingpower.org, Growing Healthy Food, People & Community
Food Corps- wwwfoodcorps.org All children know what healthy food is.
Jane Goodall- www.janegoodall.org Make a difference for all living things

~~~ ~

"I'd like to see Homo sapiens use our enormous brainpower, goodness of heart and strength of will to pull back the reins on the environmental catastrophe's that would spell our demise. We have the imagination and intelligence to create a sustainable world. A large piece of the puzzle involves major changes in the foods we cultivate and consume. As we change our diets in a radical way we will change our own health in a similarly extreme fashion. From there, the microcosm of each person's health will translate to the health of the planet." -David Sandoval

~~~~

Health Centers

Optimum Health Institute- (San Diego, California and Austin, Texas) In this holistic healing program, participants cleanse and nourish the body with diet, fasting, and exercise; quiet and focus the mind with journaling and meditation. At OHI, participants can learn how to relax, develop a positive attitude, and focus on what matters most to achieve a happy, fulfilling, and healthy life. Wheatgrass juice is consumed twice daily to cleanse cells and purify blood. Enemas and wheatgrass implants help to cleanse the colon while gentle exercise supports cleansing the lymphatic system. Hippocrates, known as the "father of medicine," taught that wholesome, natural food could help restore physical health. Healthy meals in purest form – fresh, certified-organic, and raw.

Dr. Leigh Erin Connealy MD.- Oasis of Hope, Center for New Medicine
Dr. Connealy completed her post-graduate training at the Harbor, UCLA Medical Center in Los Angeles, California. She soon realized that conventional medicine had very limited returns and did not always improve the health of her patients, who were hungry for alternative approaches to improve their health. This led her to study integrative and complementary therapies, and since then she has revolutionized the landscape of medicine.

She has discovered that many factors contribute to the disease process; therefore, many modalities must be used to reverse it. Dr. Connealy treats the WHOLE person, and is open to all potential treatment possibilities. She has over twenty years of experience in finding the 'root cause of an illness', and has taken numerous advanced courses, including homeopathic, nutritional and lifestyle approaches, while studying disease, chronic illness, and cancer treatments.

Dr. Connealy has been asked to lecture on numerous subjects and to educate other medical professionals on her findings throughout the years. She has a true passion to change her patients' health, and give them a new lease on life. Center for New Medicine www.cfnmedicine.com

Center for New Medicine- Cancer Center for Hope previously Oasis of Hope, California. In November of 2009 Cancer Center for Hope, previously Oasis of Hope California opened its first treatment center at Center For New Medicine in Irvine, California. Since then, the center has been providing world-class integrative medical cancer treatment without having to travel outside the US. The focus of Cancer Center for Hope is to treat the whole person - to look for the root cause of their cancer, including genetic, physiological, environmental, nutritional, social, emotional and spiritual factors. Cancer Center for Hope offers unique genetic testing and treatments, individualized to each patient.

Hippocrates Institute- Resting amongst 50 acres of tropical woodlands in Southern Florida, Hippocrates offers a serene setting in which to heal, nurture and develop into one's fullest potential. The Institute's signature Life Transformation Program provides the fundamental training and a definitive blueprint for transitioning to a healthier lifestyle. The Life Transformation Program is a three-week residential holistic approach program to health and wellness, where participants are taught transformation of the mind, body and spirit.

The goal of the Institute is to assist people in taking responsibility for their lives and to help them internalize and actualize an existence free from premature aging, disease and needless pain. Good health is our most prized possession, generating a positive mindset of confidence, enthusiasm, strength and joyfulness that can trigger a life of optimum achievement. At Hippocrates, the team of caregivers strives to give each and every guest the tools they need to learn how to help them help themselves.

Brian Clement- www.TheRealTruthabout Health.com In response to growing public demand for the real truth about health, nutrition and environmental information, Dr. Brian Clement produced this website to share the information and knowledge he has learned over the last 40 years. In1980, Brian assumed the title of Director of Hippocrates Health Institute and, in 1987, he moved the Institute to Florida. Since that time, he has directed the Institute's growth and development, and facilitated the implementation of progressive natural health treatments/programs.

Brian's progressive ideas on natural health, coupled with his vast theoretical and practical science experience, have provided him with the opportunity to conduct countless seminars, lectures and educational programs. He has traveled to more than 25 countries motivating the public to take action to improve their lives. Brian has also written numerous books in which he explores the various aspects of health, spirituality and natural healing including his best-selling book, "Living Foods for Optimum Health," heralded by Coretta Scott King as a "landmark guide to the essentials of healthy living."

TrueNorth Health Center was founded in 1984 by Dr. Alan Goldhamer and Dr. Jennifer Marano. The integrative medicine approach they established offers participants the opportunity to obtain evaluation and treatment for a wide variety of problems. The staff at TrueNorth Health Center includes medical doctors, osteopaths, chiropractors, naturopaths, psychologists, research scientists, and other health professionals. The Center is now the largest facility in the world that specializes in medically supervised water-only fasting.

Dr Robin Chutkan- www.digestivecenterforwomen.com. Her primarily plant-based diet, Vinyasa yoga practice and long-distance running are the foundation of her own healthy regimen and she strives to highlight the importance of nutrition, exercise and leisure to her patients.

A member of the faculty at Georgetown Hospital since 1997, Dr Chutkan founded the Digestive Center for Women (DCW) in 2004, an integrative gastroenterology practice that includes nutritional therapy and stress reducing techniques In addition to digestive disorders in women, her clinical areas of interest include alterations in gut bacteria (dysbiosis), inflammatory bowel diseases, irritable bowel syndrome, and food as medicine.

She is a recognized leader in gastroenterology both nationally and internationally and Washingtonian magazine has consistently named her one of the top doctors in her field. She is the author of the bestselling book Gutbliss, and the newly released The Microbiome Solution, and has lectured extensively throughout the United States and Europe.

Mental Health

Dr. Hyla Cass is a nationally acclaimed innovator and expert in the fields of integrative medicine, psychiatry, and addiction recovery. Dr. Cass helps individuals to take charge of their health including help for withdrawing from both psychiatric medication and substances of abuse, with the aid of natural supplements.

Dr. Cass appears often as a guest on national radio and television, including *The Dr. Oz Show, Entertainment*, and *The View*, and in national print media. She has been quoted in many national magazines, blogs for the *Huffington Post*, and is the author of several best-selling books including: *What Your Doctor Doesn't Know About Nutrition*, and *The Addicted Brain and How to Break Free*.

The concept of doctor as authority figure is replaced with a more progressive view of doctor as health partner. Dr. Cass ascribes to the following principles:

A. Treat the whole person – mind, body, spirit, and environment.
B. Determine the root causes of symptoms, using scientific lab testing if needed.
C. Apply a continuum of treatments, always beginning with the safest and most natural as possible.
She believes, that in this way, we have the opportunity to help heal our health care system, our communities, our planet, and ultimately, ourselves.

Dr. Kelly Brogan is boarded in Psychiatry, Psychosomatic Medicine, Reproductive Psychiatry, Integrative Holistic Medicine, and practices Functional Medicine, a root-cause approach to illness as a manifestation of multiple, interrelated systems. After studying Cognitive Neuroscience at M.I.T. and receiving her M.D. from Cornell University, she completed her residency and fellowship at Bellevue, NYU.

She is one of the nation's only physicians with perinatal psychiatric training who takes a holistic evidence-based approach in the care of patients, with a focus on environmental medicine and nutrition. She is also a mom of two, and an active supporter of women's birth experience, rights to birth empowerment, and limiting of unnecessary interventions. She practices in New York City.
Her focus is:
A. The danger of psychiatry and a better model of mental illness
B. Bodily problems that masquerade as psychiatric symptoms
C. Top lifestyle interventions and powerful natural treatments
D. Misconceptions around causes of mental illness
Holistic women's health psychiatry focused on the identification of root causes of symptoms and natural treatments for whole body wellness.

Julie Matthews is a Certified Nutrition Consultant specializing in autism spectrum disorders, ADHD, and nutrition for pregnancy. Her approached is based on the Bio-Individual NutritionTM needs of each person. She provides dietary guidance backed by scientific research and applied clinical experience. Her award winning book, Nourishing Hope for Autism, has helped people around the world to make food and nutrition choices that aid the health, learning, and behavior of those with autism, ADHD, and other developmental delays.

She presents at leading autism conferences in the US and abroad, and is the Nutrition Editor of the Autism File magazine. She is the co-founder of Nourishing Hope and the Bio-Individual Nutrition Institute. Julie has a private nutrition practice in San Francisco, California, and supports families and clinicians from around the world with her nutritional guidance and understanding of how the body and brain are connected.
Visit NourishingHope.com and BioIndividualNutrition.com

Sustainability, Ecological and Environmental Action

Andrew Harvey.net- Sacred Activism- This culmination of award-winning author Andrew Harvey's life's work bridges the great divide between spiritual resignation and engaged spiritual activism. A manifesto for the transformation of the world through the fusion of deep mystical peace with the clarity of radical wisdom, it is a wake-up call to put love and compassion to urgent, focused action. According to Harvey, we are in a massive global crisis reflected by a mass media addicted to violence and trivialization, at a moment when what the world actually needs is profound inspiration, a return to the heart-centered way of the Divine Feminine, take to heart the words of the mystics throughout the ages, and the cultivation of the nonviolent philosophies of Gandhi, Nelson Mandela, Aung San Suu Kyi, and the Dalai Lama.

Fair World Project (FWP) www.fairworldproject.org is an independent campaign of the Organic Consumers Association which seeks to protect the use of the term "fair trade" in the marketplace, expand markets for authentic fair trade, educate consumers about key issues in trade and agriculture, advocate for policies leading to a just economy, and facilitate collaborative relationships to create true system change. Fair World Project (FWP) educates and advocates for a just global economy where: people are treated fairly with dignity; the environment is respected and nourished; commerce fosters sustainable livelihoods and communities in a global society based on cooperation and solidarity.

Fooddemocracynow.org- Amy Harmon, Andrew Polack Food Democracy Now! A grassroots movement of more than 650,000 farmers and citizens dedicated to building a sustainable food system that protects our natural environment, sustains farmers and nourishes families. Our food system is fundamentally broken. A few companies dominate the market, prioritizing profits over people and our planet. Government policies put the interests of corporate agribusiness over the livelihoods of farm families.

Center for Food Safety- (CFS) www.Centerforfoodsafety.org is a national non-profit public interest and environmental advocacy organization working to protect human health and the environment by curbing the use of harmful food production technologies and by promoting organic and other forms of sustainable agriculture. CFS also educates consumers concerning the definition of organic food and products. CFS uses legal actions, groundbreaking scientific and policy reports, books and other educational materials, market pressure and grass roots campaigns through the True Food Network.

World Business Academy- Worldbusiness.org A non-profit think tank and network founded in 1987 with the mission to educate and inspire business leaders to take responsibility for the planetary whole. The World Business Academy is an action incubator and network of business and thought leaders. Our Mission is to inspire business to assume responsibility for the whole of society and assist those in business who share our values.

"The best of the mystic is the connection with Divine truth, power, peace and passion. And the very best of the activist is the passion to see justice done, to see the forests whole again, to see the poor fed, to see the devastating corrupt systems unravel and more just systems put in their place -- and to see humanity live in harmony with itself and our world. When you marry the fire of the mystic's passion for God, with the noblest part of the activist's longing - the fire of the

passion for justice - those two flames come together and there is a sacred alchemical reaction in the depths of our being that births a third flame, which is the flame of pure love and wisdom in action." -Andrew Harvey, Sacred Activism

Epilogue- One Way Home

I have come to realize the choice to embrace healing, to choose life, to grow our authenticity and the integral core values, exemplified in all Wisdom Traditions, though fraught with difficulty is the only real choice worth living from. For as we come to completion of our time here and look back, will we appreciate the service, the love and loved ones, and the addition we have brought to our world or look back with regret for having missed our boat and bought into ignorance and the materialistic self-indulgence of Mayas illusion, Samsara Matrix.

As I arrive at this final phase of completing Longevity Source a reoccurring dream and vision appears, taking me to depths of heart-opening feeling, along with grieving for the suffering, so prevalent on many levels. Also within this overwhelming, heart opening sadness, what has become apparent is unimagined depths of compassion, connection to Mother Earth and an exquisite appreciation for moments of seeing the incredible beauty in the minutest parts of her vast web of life. Also a tremendous gratitude for those fellow beings choosing to wake up, choosing love, choosing to join the wave of coherent resonance, choosing to make a difference and unify no matter how difficult or hopeless it looks.

This heartfelt dream and vision arrived, in part, as an inspiration and out-picturing of the name and vision of "Under the Bodhi Tree" miraculously becoming very prominent to me. Recently, my now esteemed friend and colleague, plant strong Chef Stephen Rouelle, opened an extraordinary vegan, vegetarian and raw food restaurant (Under the Bodhi Tree)-Maunalani Shops, just a few doors down from where I was working.

As I was in the process of finishing this book Stephen left his previous employment and opened what I consider the best restaurant on the Island. (Other wonderful vegan-veg cafes on the Island include; The Sweet Cane-Hilo, Sea Dandelion-Honokaa, Sweet Potato-Hawi, Ai Pono-Kona, Phresh-Kainaliu, S.Kona and Kaya's-Honalu, S.Kona).

Chef Stephen had major health and weight problems while being a head chef at a nearby luxury hotel. Upon being introduced to and embracing a vegan diet, he had lost over a hundred pounds, gained his health and became well educated to the best in vegan foods and superfoods, sustainability and responsible lifestyle choices. It has been an incredible miracle to have so much consciousness and delicious, healthy and lovingly made food in this resort shopping setting.

In my reoccurring dream, inspired by the name and incredible miracle of this restaurant, I see Buddha, under the Bodhi Tree, as well as Christ's 40 days in the desert (or any great Saint's time of soul rebirth). I imagine a deep overwhelming grief, as a being of that capacity sees and feels, not only the worlds pain then, but is also able to know the levels of suffering, beyond fathomable, present in today's world. From my point of view I envision them having doubts whether anything they could have done or do would be of help, or of any use, and then appealing to the Divine for Grace. From this place the Divine revealed, to the Beloved Ones, the resonant heart of Love that is currently emerging forth on this planet, with all who are choosing to live in loving integrity.

These masters could hear, amongst the incredible chaos, a clearly audible and coherent, vibratory LOVE call from the ever expanding, unifying wave of consciousness and commitment to Transformation emerging now. Upon seeing and feeling the incredible love and beauty awakening also, they left the desert, got up from under the Bodhi Tree and ventured forth into the world, ready now to serve the Dharma, that was their part, to help this miraculous process unfold!

Embracing a lighter, healthier diet, multiple layers of cleansing, letting go of the many differing addictions and avoidances, making life affirming choices amongst the momentum and onslaught of so much toxicity, distraction and density is often a daunting, yet always rewarding endeavor. Our predecessors have lovingly laid down the blueprint, the integral patterns of Christ Consciousness, of Unconditional Love, all-encompassing Compassion, Harmlessness and Forgiveness. The Eightfold Path, Vedic scriptures, Essene Wisdom and all true spiritual paths emphasize the oneness, the unity and the of all of creation.

In this time, where the future of Humanity rests upon what happens in the next few years, we have been lovingly given a core structure to grow a paradigm shift. What is the possible Human/Humanity at this time on Earth? Physically, emotionally and spiritually healthy, our DNA's Telomeres re-growing, connected to each other in The Flower of Life, Chakras spinning in Harmony, unified in fully integrating this wave of Awakening through the Law of Attraction, manifesting Home! Many Blessings on our transformational journey home. – Chef Todd

The Power is Ours
Special Commentary for 2015 by Sun, Gentle World Co-Founder

As we ring out the old, tumultuous year that was 2014, it is tempting to bemoan the current state of the world, and the potential disasters we face at the hands of the powers that seem to be. But the promise of change that comes with ringing in the new demands that we put those thoughts aside, and focus instead on whatever reasons we can find to inspire our hope that somehow, 2015 will bring the changes we so desperately need. Despite the feeling of despair I see permeating our present, I find real reasons to remain hopeful !

Overall, a growing number of us are willing to look deeper inside ourselves for a greater understanding of what truly matters in this life. As we do, we are discovering that we are more similar to one another than our shallow differences had led us to believe. Although bigotry is still pandemic in our society, time is its enemy, as its strength significantly weakens with each new generation. Although war is still too often the method of choice in settling disputes, many more of us question the notion that violence can ever bring about peace.

Exemplary of our deepening and expanding compassion is the rising tide of vegans who have withdrawn their support of the holocaust that is the animal industry. Virtually unchallenged for centuries, this horrific business, is, in this one, on the defensive, as we are, slowly but surely, losing our taste for enslaving, eating and using the bodies of our fellow animals.

As insane as individual human behavior still appears, there is little doubt in my mind that, as a species, we are evolving. Preposterous, frightening, disempowering beliefs that were accepted as truths without question not so long ago, are now openly debated and are ultimately being exposed as the sham they have always been. In their place has come a new understanding that the power to change the nature of our outer world is ours, with our willingness to change the nature inside us. And it is this understanding that is my greatest hope for rescuing the life of the 21st century.

We are seeing, as though with new eyes, that each of us has a unique viewing of the mystery that is the world we inhabit, and because we assume that the way we see it is reality, we live our lives as though it is. However, since our perceptions are determined by our point of view, which includes where we are standing and the direction in which we are faced, both of which are in our power to change, each and every one of us is empowered to evolve our world, simply (if not always easily) by standing for what is right, with our faces to the light.

If we want an honest world, we must live and speak what we know to be true. If we want a just world, we must be fair in all our dealings. If we want a gentle world, we must reject violence. If we want a free world, we must be willing to free our human and non-human slaves. And if we want a peaceful world, we must first find a way to make peace with ourselves and one another.

As we stand on the brink of 2015, I say to you, our readers, and to myself, in one breath: Let's make the coming year the most evolutionary in the history of the human race, because we can. With love from the Gentle World team, www.gentleworld.org.

Cover Art

Accented at the end of the DNA strand on the cover are *Telomeres*. These are the recently discovered (receiving the Nobel Prize) biological time clocks at the end of chromosomes. Every time a cell divides, it loses a piece of this "time clock" and the life of the cell shortens - thus shortening one's life! Most human cells have the potential to live a lot longer than they live which is directly related to the expression of the telomerase enzyme that is present in almost all cells, but has "turned off." Diet and lifestyle factors (Epigenetics) have been proven, by extensive testing in Dr. Dean Ornish's Lifestyle Program, to increase Telomere lengths, turning off disease genes while turning on healthy genes!

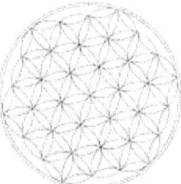

"The Flower of Life" is considered to be sacred geometry, containing ancient spiritual value, which depicts the fundamental forms of space and time. In this sense, it is believed to contain a type of basic information of all living things and is the visual expression of the connections of life that run through all sentient beings. In Esoteric thought, the Flower of Life has provided what is considered to be deep spiritual meaning and forms of enlightenment to those who have studied it, as sacred unifying geometry.

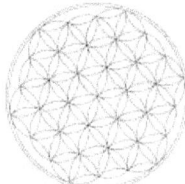

These seven chakra (pronounced chukra) symbols represent the seven main energy centers vital to health for human beings. These chakras are like spirals of energy, each one relating to the others. When spinning in harmony, propensities for love, evolution, peace, and happiness are increased. If the energy centers become blocked or depleted, then our bodies have more difficulty functioning properly and this can lead to a variety of problems on many levels. Our wellbeing is not purely a physical issue. Many more integrative health practitioners are now treating patients in a holistic manner, recognizing that we are body, mind and spirit, and none of these areas function entirely alone. Each has an effect upon the others.

Back Cover- Pictured Dishes

Middle Top

Magical Morning L.O.V.E. (Live, Organic, Vegan, Energy Breakfast)
Garnished with Goji Berries and chopped fresh Olena
Cacao Nibs and Chlorella Tablets

Raw Kale Salad with Red Radish

Raw Vegetable Soup
Garnished with Garlic Dill Sauerkraut

Top Right

Sprouted Mung and Lentil Salad
With Cherry Tomatoes and Island Dressing

Raw Sunflower, Macadamia Nut, Curried Vegetable Pate'
With Chopped Green Onions and Cucumbers

Top Left -Todd's Dish - (Tray)
Favorite Raw Dehydrated Cookies
Sprouted Buckwheat, Fig, Sunflower Seeds, with Cacao Nibs

Todd's Shirt – Designed by Vegan Superfood Chef Todd

Inspiration from Will Tuttle www.WorldPeaceDiet.org

"Vegan Spirit"
Compassionate, Sustainable, Healthy, Peaceful
Flower of Life with OM symbol on Earth
Babies; piglet, chick, calf and lamb

See "Vegan Spirit" in full and more recipe pictures at:
www.Longevitysource.com

*"For in the degree to which we come into this realization and connect ourselves
with this infinite source, do we make it possible for the higher powers to play,
work and manifest through us."* -Ralph Waldo Trine

Aloha, the Beginning

www.ingramcontent.com/pod-product-compliance
Lightning Source LLC
Chambersburg PA
CBHW080255290526
45790CB00005B/1813